THE GOOD BOOK OF
Nutrition

AMERICAN
CANCER
SOCIETY

*A Recipe Collection and
Guide to Healthful Eating.
It's good for you!*

T he American Cancer Society, North Carolina Division, Inc., gratefully acknowledges the American Cancer Society, Florida Division, Inc., and Publix Super Markets, Inc., for making the production of this Nutritional Cookbook possible. This book was originally developed by the American Cancer Society, Florida Division, Inc., and Publix Super Markets, Inc.; David V. Schapira, M.D., H. Lee Moffitt Cancer Center, for serving as the project's medical advisor; Beatriz de Pando, R.D., clinical dietitian, and Nagi Kumar, R.D., research dietitian, H. Lee Moffitt Cancer Center; Patricia Wallden Hall, home economist; Judy McGinty, M.S., R.D. and Linda LaVine, R.D., Florida Dietetic Association; and J. Gail Vogt, director of food and nutrition services, H. Lee Moffitt Cancer Center, for spending countless hours procuring and analyzing recipes.

Publisher: Favorite Recipes Press,
    a Division of Great American Opportunities, Inc.
    P.O. Box 305142, Nashville, Tennessee 37230

Library of Congress Catalog Number: 87-28318
ISBN: 0-87197-223-9

Manufactured in the United States of America

First Printing 90,000 copies, 1987
Second Printing 20,000 copies, 1988
Third Printing 17,000 copies, 1988
Fourth Printing 8,000 copies, 1988
Fifth Printing 25,000 copies, 1988

Contents

While studies have shown an important relationship between diet and the risk of developing cancer, following the recipes and nutritional guidelines included in this book does not guarantee prevention of the disease. It is important to have regular checkups and see your doctor immediately if you think that you might have cancer.

The American Cancer Society is the largest voluntary health organization in the United States. Through a corps of 2.5 million volunteers, the Society is committed to eradicating cancer and to improving the quality of life for cancer patients. These goals are accomplished through a three-fold program of research, health education and patient assistance.

Research

The American Cancer Society is the largest source of private cancer research funds nationally, with its overall investment climbing from $1 million in 1946 to $82 million in 1987. The Society places grants where volunteer leadership feels the most innovative and promising research ideas are being explored.

Education

Educating the public about ways of preventing or reducing one's cancer risk is an important focus of the ACS. Target areas include the relationship between diet, nutrition and cancer as well as smoking. The value of periodic, cancer-related checkups and specific cancer tests is also stressed.

The majority of cancer cases involve colon/rectum, breast, lung, uterus, oral cavity and skin. The ACS conducts programs on all of these sites and other cancer-related topics at no charge.

Professional education keeps physicians, nurses, dentists and allied health professionals up-to-date on the latest trends in cancer research, treatment and diagnosis. Conferences on these subjects are continually planned as an integral part of the ACS educational effort.

Patient Assistance And Rehabilitation

Service and rehabilitation programs offer information, guidance and support both for cancer patients and their families. Trained ACS volunteers play an important role by participating in pre- and post-operative support programs for those directly and indirectly affected by cancer.

ACS special programs include:

CanSurmount: a short-term visitation program for patients and family members involving ACS representatives who have had the same type of cancer.

I Can Cope: an eight-week series of classes addressing the day-to-day issues facing cancer patients, their families and close friends.

Reach to Recovery: a visitation program providing support and guidance to breast cancer patients.

The ACS also provides such services as transportation to hospitals and doctors' offices, in-home care, equipment loans and much more.

EXPENDITURES FOR THE YEAR
ENDED AUGUST 31, 1987

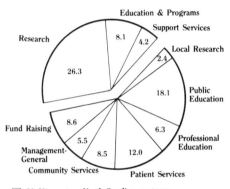

□ 61.4% spent on North Carolina programs
□ 38.6% allocated to National Office for research, program development and general supporting services.

Looking Back, Looking Forward

The ACS has seen remarkable strides made in saving lives and in increasing public awareness of steps which can be taken to protect against cancer. Through volunteers, we have raised the level of hope and inspiration. The ACS continues to advance toward its ultimate objective of a world free of cancer. We are proud of the confidence which our communities have placed in us. We are *your* American Cancer Society.

* *A detailed financial report is available by contacting your local American Cancer Society office.*

The next time you stand in the checkout line at the supermarket, look at the persons in front of and behind you. Statistically, one of the three of you will get cancer.

According to the American Cancer Society, the chances of developing cancer are rising each year. The likelihood that an American would develop cancer was 30% in 1970. It had risen to 35% in 1985 and it will rise to 40% in the year 2000.

It is not inevitable that we get cancer. In fact it is thought that by making certain changes in our lifestyle, we can greatly reduce or delay the likelihood of developing cancer. It is estimated that 75% of all cancers are potentially preventable. This information is based on the fact that people in other parts of the world have much lower cancer rates than the cancer rates in the United States.

The breast cancer rate is 6 times lower in Japan than in the U.S.; the prostate cancer rate is 125 times lower in Shanghai; and the uterine (womb) cancer rate is 40 times lower in Japan. When the Japanese moved to the United States at the turn of the century, they developed the same incidence of cancer that was prevailing in the U.S. Therefore, the cancers were not due to differences in genes or heredity.

We tend to feel that we do not have a great deal of control over our health, particularly serious illnesses like cancer, heart attacks or strokes.

The fact is that we can have a great deal of control over our health—if we choose. The most important factor that actually determines whether we develop cancer, heart attacks or strokes is what we eat. Diet is probably responsible for 35% of all cancers. The main factors thought to cause cancer include: Diet 35%, Smoking 30%, Infection 10%, Sunlight 8%, Alcohol 5%, Family History 2%, Pollution 2%, Radiation 2%, and Food Additives 1%. (Doll, R. and Peto, R. *The causes of cancer: Quantitative estimates of available risks of cancer in the United States today.* J. Nat. Can. Inst. 66: 1192-11308, 1981)

Cancer research has shown that dietary factors probably account for over one third of all the cancers we develop. Eating too many calories or too much fat has been linked to the development of five of the six most common cancers—cancers of the breast, colon, pancreas, prostate and uterus (womb). Eating too much fat has also been linked to hardening of the arteries, which can cause heart attacks and strokes.

As the food that we eat can be so important in determining whether we develop these diseases, it makes good sense to learn more about food and, if necessary, to make some changes. These changes still allow you to shop in the same places and eat in the same restaurants. You just make alterations in what food you buy and how you prepare it. You can still enjoy the food. This is the reason that this cookbook was written. Cooking in a healthy way can be tasty and easy. When you begin making changes in the food you eat and how you cook, you will see that it is not difficult. We also want to show you that shopping for foods that are healthier is not difficult.

Obstacles That Prevent Change

There are three important obstacles that prevent us from altering our lifestyles so that we reduce our risk of developing cancer, a heart attack or a stroke.

Most of us think that we are at less risk of developing these diseases than our peers. Because we are human, we tend to think "not me" when relating to our risk of developing cancer. This protection of self-esteem can blind us to the need for lifestyle change.

We tend to blame the causes of these diseases on factors that are out of our control, so that when we develop them, we don't blame ourselves. The factors that cause cancer are very much under our control. Dietary factors, smoking and sunlight probably account for the development of almost 75% of all cancers. The factors beyond our control that we like to blame are much less important. Our family history, food additives, pollution and radiation altogether contribute to less than 10% of all cancers.

Even if we wanted to eat healthily, it is difficult to know how to translate the recommendations into practical choices in the supermarket and when we eat out. In a recent study, we found that fewer than 5% of the people knew how much fat, fiber, vitamin A, calcium or salt they should eat in a day. However, a large proportion of people said they read food labels.

Motivating Change

Not only do we have to make the knowledge of how to eat healthily easy to understand and implement, we should also make these healthy choices attractive. Touting foods as nutritious or healthy may not inspire most people to buy them. An example from *Advertising Age* magazine demonstrates a clever way to market a health food.

A serpent in the Garden of Eden had something called an apple that he wanted Eve to sample. Being in the Garden of Eden, she was already surrounded by all kinds of temptations. He slithered up to her, stuck it under her nose, and said, "Try this." She jumped back and said, "What is it?"

The serpent launched into his sales pitch. "It's a fruit. It grows on the Tree of Paradise and it's mostly roughage, so it's good for your colon. It's a product of nature, 85% water with vitamins A and C, calcium, thiamine, riboflavin and iron."

Eve said, "I've never heard of vitamins and my colon is fine," and promptly made her way to the premium ice cream shop.

The serpent was discouraged but he decided to give it another shot.

Assuming that Eve was in a family-sized household, the serpent approached Eve and said, "Psst, Mom, try this! It's a fruit called the apple and your kids are going to love it. It's sweet, crunchy, great for after-school energy and doesn't cause cavities."

Eve said, "Forget it. Cain and Abel have enough energy. They're killing each other already," and she turned on her heel.

The snake was crushed. He thought for days. Finally he decided on one last-ditch effort to sell his apple. He polished the apple until it glistened in the sun and hung it on a tree where Eve could not miss it. Then he crawled into the bushes.

The apple suddenly caught Eve's eye, and she just had to know more, so she sought out the serpent and said, "What is it?"

The snake casually said, "It's new. It's a tempting dessert. It's sinful and all natural. It's very indulgent and low in calories. It's called 'Fatal Apple,' and you probably can't afford it."

Eve replied, "Says who? I'll take a bushel."

CARCINOGENESIS
Converting a Normal Cell to a Cancer Cell
To understand why most cancers are preventable, it is important to know how a normal cell is converted to a cancer cell. There are two stages to the carcinogenic process: Initiation and Promotion.

Initiation is a one-time, irreversible event. When a normal cell is initiated, it is primed to become a cancer cell but cannot be converted to a cancer cell unless it is exposed to a promoter.

Promotion is the second essential step in carcinogenesis. The primed initiated cell is exposed to a promoter. After several years of exposure to a promoter, the initiated cell converts to a cancer cell.

To convert a normal cell to a cancer cell, two mistakes have to occur at exactly the right locations in the genetic material—DNA—in our cells. DNA is like a stepladder, where every group of rungs is a gene. Let us say that to produce cancer, the mistakes need to occur at rungs number 27 and 53. Initiation will produce the first error at rung 27. If only a few cells in our body had the one mistake at rung 27, then the chances of a second mistake's occurring at exactly the correct point in the DNA, rung 53, would be extremely small. If we produce millions of copies of the cell with the one mistake at rung 27, the chances of getting the second mistake at rung 53 are much higher.

Initiated cells appear normal, but they are different from normal cells in one important respect—they can divide more quickly than normal cells if they are exposed to a promoter. Two promoters that we are aware of are dietary fat and cigarette smoke. By stimulating initiated cells to divide more rapidly than normal, a promoter will produce millions more copies of the initiated cell with the one DNA error. This greatly increases the chances of a second error's occurring at exactly the right location in the DNA—at rung number 53. The lower the concentration of promoter the initiated cell is exposed to and the briefer the time of exposure, the less proliferation of initiated cells there will be, and, therefore, the less chance there will be for a cancer cell to develop.

PREVENTING CANCER

It is intervening in the process of promotion that holds the promise for preventing or delaying the occurrence of cancer. An excellent example of this principle is cigarette smoking. The main carcinogens in cigarette smoke are both initiators and promoters. If a person stops smoking, initiated cells in the lining of the lung are no longer exposed to the promotional effects of cigarette smoke. The risk of lung cancer in ex-smokers starts falling after the first year and after 7 to 8 years of cessation is almost the same as someone who never has smoked a cigarette in his life.

Fat

The average Japanese person obtains only 25% of all the calories eaten in a day from fat. The average American person obtains 42% of daily calories from fat. The Japanese adopted American eating habits and ate more fat after they moved to the U.S. In fact, with the increase in Western-style restaurants in Japan, the fat consumption has increased over the past 25 years and so has their incidence of breast cancer.

Animals that are fed a high-fat or a high-calorie diet develop more cancers of the breast and colon compared to animals fed a low-fat diet. If the animals fed the high-fat diet are changed to a low-fat diet the incidence of tumors decreases.

Vitamin A

Vitamin A that comes from the diet ensures the normal growth of the cells that line the esophagus (gullet), lung, cervix and bladder. Studies have shown that people who eat a diet low in vitamin A have a high incidence of these cancers when compared to people who eat a diet rich in vitamin A. We would like to stress that this protective effect of vitamin A comes from dietary sources, not vitamin pills. The vitamin A from pills is not protective and can be stored in the liver and cause liver damage.

Fiber

Populations that eat food that is high in fiber have a lower incidence of cancer of the colon, the second most common cancer in the United States. This decrease in incidence is even greater if the high-fiber intake is combined with a low-fat intake. The fiber changes the bacteria in the colon from bacteria that produce carcinogens to those that decrease the production. The bacteria that produce carcinogens thrive in the absence of oxygen. When we eat fiber, it ferments and produces oxygen, which decreases the number of those carcinogen-producing bacteria present.

AMERICAN CANCER SOCIETY RECOMMENDATIONS

Based on current scientific knowledge the American Cancer Society recommends that a person should:

• Decrease his dietary fat intake to 30% or less of the total calories he consumes in a day.

• Increase his intake of green and yellow vegetables which are rich in vitamin A and increase his intake of cruciferous vegetables (cabbage, cauliflower, Brussels sprouts) which contain substances that neutralize carcinogens in our bodies.

• Increase his intake of dietary fiber to 25 to 30 grams per day.

OBESITY AND FAD DIETS
The Rhythm Method of Girth Control

There is another important reason why it's important to know what you are eating—weight control. An American Cancer Society study showed that people who were more than 40% overweight increased their risk of cancer of the colon, breast, prostate, gall bladder, ovary and uterus. As you read this, over 65 million fellow Americans will be on a diet trying to lose weight. In just a fifteen-year period from the early 1960's to the late 1970's, the average weight of the American man increased by 6 pounds and the average weight of the American woman increased by 4 pounds. Another important factor is what effect our eating habits have on our children. Federal nutrition surveys have shown that obesity among American children six to eleven years old has increased 54% in the past two decades. What are our chances of reversing this trend? The success rate of all weight-loss programs in this country is 5% at one year. Clearly, what has been shown is that losing weight rapidly on a diet program not only does not work for very long, but even worse, it alters the composition of your body and your metabolism.

When you lose weight rapidly, you lose mainly water during the first ten days. You then break down muscle as a source of calories to compensate for your reduced-calorie intake. Finally, after about two weeks, you break down fat and decrease the amount of fat on the body. When people lose weight rapidly, they decrease the amount of lean body mass. When they regain weight, they just gain fat which again decreases the percentage of lean body mass. This repeated rapid weight loss and the regaining of weight is called the "rhythm method of girth control." The changing of body composition to increase the amount of fat and decrease the amount of muscle lowers metabolism. Each time a person loses and then gains weight, the next time he attempts to lose weight he has to eat fewer calories than during the previous attempt, and it takes longer to lose the same amount of weight.

To successfully lose weight and maintain the loss, you must make changes slowly so that your palate adjusts to the change, and you do not want to eat the high-fat foods you ate previously.

MAKING SENSE OF CALORIES
Fat and Food Labeling

If we are going to eat less fat and fewer calories, we should be able to identify which foods are high in fat and either eat less of them or choose alternatives that are lower in fat. To simplify this complicated area, we need just a few facts.

The American Cancer Society recommends that only 30% of all the calories we eat in a day should come from fat. The average recommended allowances of calories and fat for the average man and woman are listed below.

DAILY CALORIE AND FAT INTAKE FOR THE AVERAGE MAN AND WOMAN

	Man	Woman
Calories	2100	1700
Grams fat	70	55

Obviously, people vary in size, level of activity and calories they burn, but this generalization will give you some idea how high in fat and calories certain foods can be.

READING A FOOD LABEL

When you look at a food label, look at two important items: the calories per serving and grams of fat. A simple manipulation will translate those values into more useful information—what percentage of the product is fat.

Learning this calculation will allow you to evaluate whether the food item identified as lower in fat is indeed low in fat. When a product is identified as "90% fat-free, 10% fat," the reference is to the percentage of fat by weight. The percentage of calories that comes from fat can be as high as 50 to 60%. If you don't take the trouble to know how to calculate the percentage of calories from fat, you may be misled into thinking the product is low in fat.

Example A

Calories per serving—200

Grams of fat—5

To calculate the percentage of calories from fat in this food product you must:

1) Multiply the grams of fat by 9 (the number of calories in a gram of fat). This factor of 9 never changes.
   5 x 9 = 45

2) Divide the product in number 1 (45) by the calories per serving.
   45 ÷ 200 = 0.22

3) Multiply the answer in number 2 (0.22) by 100 to convert to percent of calories from fat.
   0.22 x 100 = 22%

This is the percent of calories in this food product that comes from fat.

Example B

Calories per serving = 50
     Grams of fat = 4

1) Multiply grams of fat x 9
   4 x 9 = 36
2) Divide product by calories per
   serving   36 ÷ 50 = 0.72
3) Multiply by 100 to get calories
   from fat   0.72 x 100 = 72%

SIMPLE WAYS TO CUT CALORIES AND FAT

When you cut down the amount of fat in the food you eat, you should retrain your palate slowly. When you eat fat, it distends the stomach by slowing down its emptying and makes you feel bloated. The distension of the stomach stimulates the production of endorphins, the body's own natural morphine, which gives you that tired, sleepy feeling after a big, fatty meal. By eating lower fat foods, you can avoid this unpleasant feeling and have better control over your weight. The following changes can be made while still shopping at the same supermarket and eating in the same restaurants.

A simple way to cut fat and calories when you cook a meal is to use herbs and spices to flavor the meal instead of butter. If you don't have herbs, get a friend to lend you some and live off borrowed thyme.

Meat

If you eat red meat, reduce the frequency to 2 to 3 times per week. Buy lean cuts, and trim the visible fat off. Trimming off the visible fat reduces the fat and calorie content by half. Sausage and pork are very high in fat and calories. Luncheon meats that come from turkey are lower in fat.

Eat more poultry. It is lower in fat. When you buy poultry, take the skin off before you cook it. A chicken provides about 2000 calories. If you take the skin off before cooking, you will reduce the calorie content to 600 calories. If you take the skin off after cooking the chicken, the calorie content is 1300 calories. Deep-frying poultry greatly increases the fat and calorie content. A deep-fried chicken wing and thigh (with the skin on) contains 48 grams of fat (almost a day's fat for a woman) and 810 calories.

When meat is put on the barbecue, fat drips on to the coals and is burnt as pyrrolated hydrocarbons. These are deposited on the steak and are equivalent to the carcinogens in 600 cigarettes. To decrease this deposition, cook lower fat foods, put foil on the grill and avoid flames developing on the coals. The high intake of smoked and salted foods is why stomach cancer is much more common among the Japanese.

Fish

Eat more fish as it is low in fat. The oils in fish are thought to be responsible for the low incidence of heart attacks among the Eskimos. The oil thought to produce this effect is eicosapentaenoic acid or E.P.A. In order for Americans to eat amounts of E.P.A. equivalent to that of the Eskimos, we would have to eat fish almost all day, because the type of fish we eat is much lower in E.P.A. As this substance prolongs the time the blood takes to clot, one must be careful taking a fish oil supplement, which at this time cannot be recommended.

When you cook fish, broil, bake or poach it, and season it with lemon juice, garlic, pepper or salt (or salt substitute) rather than adding butter. If you buy canned fish, buy the water-packed variety which has 5 to 10 times less fat than the oil-packed variety.

Although fish contains less fat than red meat, the cholesterol content in certain shellfish can be high. Oysters and lobster contain over 200 milligrams of cholesterol per serving. The American Heart Association recommends limiting the consumption of cholesterol to 300 milligrams per day to prevent heart disease and strokes.

Dairy Products

Drink milk that is low in fat. The label can be misleading. The following list gives the fat content of milk products.

Dairy Product	Percent Calories from Fat
Half and Half	80
Whole Milk	48
2% Milk	37
1% Buttermilk	20
1% Milk	18
Skim Milk	5

If you currently drink whole milk, change gradually by switching to 2% and then 1%. Most people who switch to 1% or skim milk don't switch back to the creamy taste of whole milk.

Eat low-fat cheeses and low-fat yogurt. Most regular cheeses have 60 to 70% calories from fat. Low-fat cottage and mozzarella cheeses are low in fat. Low-fat yogurts can also be used to make dips.

Eat desserts that are low in fat. Sorbet contains no fat and is 80 calories per serving. Low-fat ice milk, sherbet or frozen yogurt are low in fat and usually lower in calories. Two scoops of these products contain about 200 calories and 6 grams of fat. Two scoops of ice cream can contain as many as 600 calories and 35 grams of fat. The percentage of milk fat in ice cream varies greatly among brands.

Salads and Soups

Buy low-calorie and low-fat salad dressings. When you pour a ladle (2 ounces) of regular salad dressing on your salad, you are placing the equivalent of a cheeseburger and four teaspoons of sugar on your salad. Most people use 3 to 4 ounces of dressing—two cheeseburgers and eight teaspoons of sugar on their salad. Buy "lite" mayonnaise which has ⅓ less fat. You probably couldn't tell the difference between "lite" and the regular mayonnaise on a sandwich.

One study showed that the calorie content on the plate of the people who had a salad from a salad bar was 1,000. With salad dressing, bacon bits, ham and cheese, the fat and calories can add up. Don't build huge salads and cover them with rich high-calorie, high-fat salad dressing.

Soup can be filling, replace a meal, and be very low in fat. Lentil or bean, vegetable or chicken and rice soups are low in fat. If you're still hungry eat a salad with low-fat dressing. The whole meal will be very low in fat.

Snacks

Nuts are very high in fat. A handful of peanuts (3.5 ounces) has over 600 calories and contains a day's fat requirement for a woman. Eating three handfuls of peanuts means you shouldn't eat anything else all day and absolutely no fat for the next three days.

Buy low-fat potato chips, or eat pretzels. Regular potato chips are 60% fat. Donuts are high in fat, and the sugar raises your insulin level which increases hunger. Needless to say, chocolate is high in fat.

Fast or "Sudden" Food

Some of the meals that you can buy in a fast food restaurant can be so high in fat and calories that we call them "sudden" food. Sudden food is even faster than fast food. When you order a meal in these restaurants, you can consume more than the calories and fat required for a day suddenly in one sitting.

This means you don't need to eat any other meals that day and will, therefore, have plenty of time for other activities. This type of meal would consist of a double cheeseburger, fries and a regular chocolate milkshake—1500 calories and 60 grams of fat. If you eat in a fast food restaurant, be aware that the meal you eat could be more than your calorie and fat requirements for the whole day.

INCREASING YOUR DIETARY VITAMIN A INTAKE

The daily requirement of dietary vitamin A is 5,000 International Units (I.U.). Green and yellow vegetables are high in vitamin A. For instance, when eating a salad, choose the dark green lettuce as opposed to the iceberg lettuce, which is low in vitamin A. The following list will give you an idea which vegetables and fruit are high in vitamin A.

Dietary vitamin A content of vegetables and fruit

½ cup	Vitamin A Content I.U.
Kale	8,900
Carrot	8,000
Turnip Greens	7,600
Spinach	6,700
Watercress	4,700
Cantaloupe	2,500
Romaine Lettuce	2,500
Tomato	2,000
Boston Bibb Lettuce	970
Iceberg Lettuce	330

The dietary vitamin A content of the recipes in this book should be increased by adding vegetables or fruit to the dish when appropriate. Vegetables should be lightly steamed. Overcooking them can reduce the vitamin A content by 30%.

For those people who like to cheat on diets, carrot cake should not be classified as a vegetable.

INCREASING YOUR FIBER INTAKE

You should try to eat 25 to 30 grams of fiber a day. A breakfast cereal can be a good source of fiber and complex carbohydrates. Cereals that are high in fiber should contain at least 7 grams of fiber per serving. The label on the front of the package can be misleading. Be sure to rely on the nutrition information panel. Bran muffins, whole wheat bread, beans, peas, raspberries, apples and pears are a good source of fiber.

REACTING TO FOOD

Does the name Pavlov ring a bell?

One of the most important ways that we can reduce the amount of fat and calories we eat is to avoid the cues that make us hungry—such as the sight or smell of food—particularly between mealtimes. When we are exposed to these cues, we become hungry, and we want to eat. The following suggestions are ways that will help you control how much food you buy and eat:

Eat slowly—you will tend to eat less. One study showed that people ate five bites of food per minute when fast music was played in the background, four bites per minute with slow music and three bites per minute with no music. Remember the magic phrase—goblin your food is bad for your elf.

Do not engage in other activities, such as watching television, while eating.

Always sit down to eat, and use eating utensils. Put the utensils down between bites. Never eat out of food containers.

When serving the family, put the food directly on the plates. Smaller plates make the meal look larger. Do not serve food in a large container that is placed in the middle of the table for each person to help himself.

Never eat leftovers when you clear up just because the food will be wasted.

Get your spouse or friends to support your dietary goals. Preferably get their participation.

When you eat out:

Be assertive. Avoid peer pressure—make your own choice.

Plan the meals away from home.

Be selective about the restaurant you choose. Make sure alternative low-fat choices are available.

Question the waiter, owner or host regarding the ingredients and the methods of preparation.

When in a restaurant, ask the waiter to put butter, salad dressing and sauces on the side of the plate.

In preparing this cookbook, the American Cancer Society has demonstrated that cooking in a healthy way can be tasty and easy. You will notice that the fat content in some of the recipes is in excess of the recommended amount. These recipes are included as the total fat content is low or the fat comes mainly from olive oil. Countries that cook with olive oil appear to have lower incidences of the common cancers, and olive oil does not seem to raise the level of cholesterol in the blood. The recipes should be served with vegetables and fruit, when appropriate, to increase the content of vitamins A and C and fiber.

It is extremely important to understand that you alone play the most important part in determining whether you develop cancer. It is never too late to make a difference. Once you start making the changes in the food you buy, what you eat away from home and how you cook, you will find these changes are not difficult to make. Start today.

David V. Schapira, M.B.Ch.B., F.R.C.P. (C) Chief, Section of Cancer Prevention, H. Lee Moffitt Cancer Center & Research Institute; Associate Professor of Medicine, Division of Medical Oncology, University of South Florida College of Medicine, Tampa.

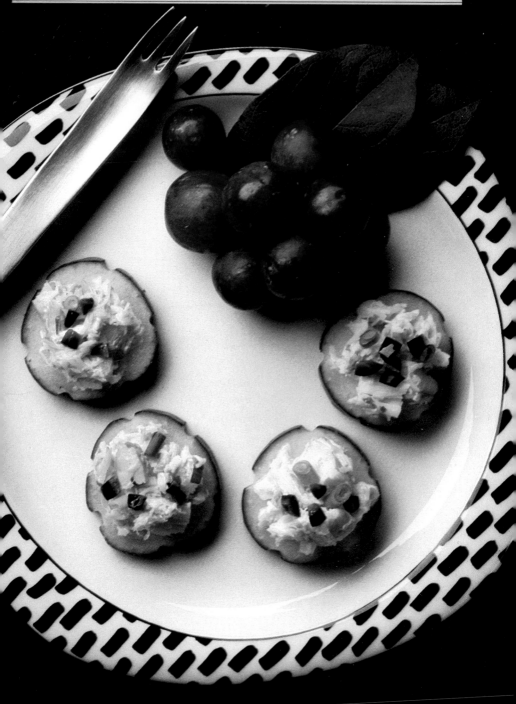

Appetizers don't have to be a threat to healthy eating if you keep a few tips in mind.

The key is to eat slowly. Hors d' oeuvres or appetizers before a dinner are meant to stimulate the appetite—not kill it!

Stay away from deep-fried foods and little tidbits laden with heavy cream.

Avoid cheese—it is usually high in fat and calories.

Avoid cheese spreads, crackers, dips and chips. Herb cream cheese spreads are very high in fat—as are the crackers you spread them on. Dips are usually made from sour cream. Try lower fat "lite" chips with a dip mixed from non-fat yogurt and low-fat cottage cheese with seasonings. Crunchy vegetables are just as satisfying, or try pretzels.

Nuts, although crammed with fat and calories, are compact sources of protein, vitamin B, vitamin E, minerals and fiber. The fat (about 50%) is primarily unsaturated, so not all bad. Dry-roasted nuts are better for you than roasted nuts which are processed in oil (usually coconut and peanut, which are saturated fats).

A handful of peanuts, a plate full of fried chicken wings, or several mini-quiches before the meal could add up to your fat and calorie allowance for that mealtime—before you sit down.

Recipe for this photograph on page 25.

CRUDITÉS WITH CREAMY DILL DIP

Prepare a colorful selection of raw vegetables: cauliflower, carrots, red, yellow and purple peppers, snow peas, baby corn, zucchini, Belgian endive, green and yellow beans, celery, fennel, cut into strips suitable for dipping. Arrange on a large platter with dip in center.

4 carrots
2 red, yellow or green
   bell peppers
½ small cauliflower
2 heads Belgian endive
¼ pound mushrooms
1 cup low-fat cottage cheese
¼ cup fresh dill, chopped or
   2 teaspoons dried dillweed
3 tablespoons low-fat
   plain yogurt
1 teaspoon fresh parsley,
   chopped
Salt and freshly ground pepper
   to taste

Cut carrots and peppers into strips. Separate cauliflower into florets. Separate endive leaves. Cut large mushrooms into halves. Chill until serving time. In a food processor container combine cottage cheese, dill, yogurt, parsley and salt and pepper. Process by pulsing until mixed. Chill in refrigerator. Around the edge of a serving platter arrange vegetables. Into a small bowl spoon dip; place in center of vegetables. Makes 10 servings.

Approx. per serving: 23.0 calories; 0.5 gr. fat; 19.56% calories from fat.

HONEY-LIME DIP FOR FRUIT

Delicious at the beginning or end of a meal, this refreshing dip can be made with lemon or lime. Choose a colorful variety of fruit: strawberries, grapes, pineapple wedges, apple, mango, papaya, pear, peach, melon, sections of orange or other seasonal fresh fruit. Arrange the fruit on a large platter with the dip in the center and let guests help themselves.

1 cup low-fat plain yogurt
2 tablespoons honey
1 tablespoon fresh lime juice
Grated rind of 1 fresh lime

In a small bowl combine yogurt, honey, lime juice and rind; mix well. Cover. Chill overnight. Into a serving bowl spoon dip. Serve with fruit. Makes 6 servings.

Approx. per serving: 57.1 calories; 0.58 gr. fat; 9.14% calories from fat.

LOW-CALORIE
SPINACH DIP

For an eye-catching centerpiece serve spinach dip in a hollowed-out red or green cabbage. An alternative to potato chips for dips is a tray full of steamed fresh artichoke leaves.

1 package (10 ounces) frozen
  chopped spinach, thawed
1 cup low-fat plain yogurt
½ cup low-fat cottage cheese
1 to 2 tablespoons 1% low-fat milk
½ cup fresh parsley, chopped
½ cup green onions, chopped
3 tablespoons lite mayonnaise
½ teaspoon (or more) fresh dill,
  minced or ¼ teaspoon
  dried dillweed
½ teaspoon seasoned salt
  (optional)
Freshly ground pepper to taste

Drain spinach well. In a medium bowl mix spinach with yogurt. In a blender container purée cottage cheese with enough milk to make of consistency of sour cream. Add to spinach mixture with parsley, green onions, mayonnaise, dill, seasoned salt and pepper; mix well. Cover. Refrigerate for 5 hours to overnight. Makes 14 (¼-cup) servings.

Approx. per serving: 33.0 calories; 1.0 gr. fat; 27.27% calories from fat.

SNAPPY
TUNA DIP

Serve with celery and carrot sticks to reduce calories and add fiber.

1 cup low-fat cottage cheese
1 can (7 ounces) water-pack tuna
Fresh lemon juice to taste
¼ teaspoon fresh dill, crushed or
  ⅛ teaspoon dried dillweed
2 green onions, sliced
Paprika to taste

In a food processor container place cottage cheese. Process until creamy. Add tuna, lemon juice and dill. Process until smooth. Stir in green onions. Into a serving bowl spoon tuna dip. Refrigerate for 1 hour or longer. Garnish with paprika. Serve with low-fat crackers or crudités. Makes 6 (¼-cup) servings.

Approx. per serving: 69.7 calories; 1.01 gr. fat; 13.04% calories from fat.

TERIYAKI
BEEF RUMAKI

Wrap tender strips of marinated beef around crunchy water chestnuts for a delectable hot appetizer.

¾ pound (½-inch thick) lean
   sirloin, round or flank steak
¼ cup lite soy sauce
1 teaspoon Worcestershire sauce
1 teaspoon onion, minced
1 teaspoon granulated sugar
1 clove garlic, minced
½ teaspoon ginger
1 can (10 ounces) water
   chestnuts

Freeze steak for 30 minutes for easier slicing. Trim off fat. Slice cross grain into about twenty-five ⅛ x 3-inch strips. In a large bowl combine soy sauce, Worcestershire sauce, onion, sugar, garlic and ginger. Add steak; stir until coated. Marinate at room temperature for 30 minutes or in refrigerator overnight, stirring occasionally. Drain. Wrap steak strip around each water chestnut; secure with toothpick. On a baking sheet arrange beef rumaki. Broil for 3 to 4 minutes or until medium-rare. (Or in a shallow glass baking dish arrange rumaki and microwave on High for 3 to 4 minutes, turning dish ¼ turn after 1½ to 2 minutes). On a serving platter arrange hot rumaki. Makes 5 servings.

Approx. per serving: 195.0 calories; 7.3 gr. fat; 33.69% calories from fat.

CHICKEN
PUFFS

These are elegant miniature chicken soufflés that are easy to prepare.

½ cup cooked boneless, skinless
   chicken, finely minced
1½ tablespoons lite mayonnaise
1 tablespoon dry bread crumbs
2 teaspoons scallions, minced
¼ teaspoon salt (optional)
¼ teaspoon dry mustard
¼ teaspoon curry powder
¼ teaspoon Worcestershire
   sauce
6 slices whole wheat bread
1 egg white
Paprika

In a large bowl combine chicken, mayonnaise, crumbs, scallions, salt, mustard, curry powder and Worcestershire sauce; mix well. Chill in refrigerator for several hours if desired. Preheat oven to 250 degrees. Cut each bread slice into 4 squares. On a baking sheet arrange bread squares. Bake for 30 minutes. In a small mixer bowl beat egg white until soft peaks form. Preheat oven to 500 degrees. Fold egg white into chicken mixture gently. Spoon onto toast squares. Sprinkle with paprika. Bake for 5 minutes. Serve immediately. Makes 24 appetizers.

Approx. per appetizer: 25.5 calories; 0.7 gr. fat; 24.7% calories from fat.

SPICED CHICKEN CUBES

½ medium onion, chopped
3 cloves garlic, minced
2 tablespoons corn oil or
    safflower oil
2 tablespoons red wine vinegar
2 tablespoons catsup
1½ teaspoons cumin, ground
1½ teaspoons paprika
2 teaspoons fresh cilantro
    (coriander), minced or
    1 teaspoon dried coriander,
    ground
¼ teaspoon ginger, ground
¼ teaspoon black pepper
⅛ teaspoon cayenne pepper
1½ pounds uncooked boneless,
    skinless chicken or turkey
    breast, cut into bite-sized pieces
2 cans (8 ounces each) whole
    water chestnuts, drained and
    cut into halves
Toothpicks
Lettuce leaves

In a medium glass bowl combine onion and garlic. Add oil, vinegar, catsup, cumin, paprika, cilantro, ginger and peppers; mix well. Add chicken; mix well. Marinate for several hours. Preheat oven to 350 degrees. Drain chicken; reserving marinade. Skewer 1 piece chicken and 1 water chestnut half onto each toothpick. In a shallow baking dish place chicken cubes. Pour reserved marinade over chicken cubes. Bake for 10 minutes; drain. On a serving plate arrange lettuce leaves. Arrange chicken on prepared plate. Makes 48 appetizers.

Approx. per appetizer: 34.4 calories; 1.1 gr. fat; 28.77% calories from fat.

BITE-SIZED SPINACH EGG FOO YUNG

5 ounces frozen chopped spinach
3 ounces egg substitute *
½ cup water chestnuts,
    finely chopped
¼ cup green bell pepper,
    finely chopped
¼ cup onion, finely chopped
¼ teaspoon salt (optional)
Dash of pepper

Cook spinach using package directions; drain. In a large bowl combine spinach, Egg Beaters, water chestnuts, green pepper, onion, salt and pepper; mix well. Preheat nonstick griddle according to manufacturer's instructions. Drop egg mixture by teaspoonfuls onto hot griddle. Cook over medium-high heat until brown on both sides. On a baking sheet place foo yung bites in single layer; cover. Chill until 30 minutes before serving time. Preheat oven to 300 degrees. Bake foo yung bites for 20 to 30 minutes or until very hot. Serve with sweet and sour sauce. Makes 36 appetizers.

* Nutritional analysis based on using *Fleischmann's Egg Beaters* egg substitute. Fat and calorie content may vary between brands.

Approx. per appetizer: 7.0 calories; 0.3 gr. fat; 38.0% calories from fat.

EGGPLANT CAVIAR

Often called "Poor Man's Caviar," this Mediterranean dip is delicious with raw vegetables or as a spread with melba toast or crackers.

1 large (1¼ pounds) eggplant
1 large tomato, peeled and
   chopped
3 green onions, finely chopped
½ stalk celery, finely chopped
¼ cup green bell pepper, minced
   (optional)
1 large clove garlic, minced
2 teaspoons corn oil or
   safflower oil
1 teaspoon fresh lemon juice
½ teaspoon salt (optional)
½ teaspoon pepper, freshly ground

Preheat oven to 400 degrees. Prick eggplant in several places with fork. On a baking sheet place eggplant. Bake for 45 minutes or until tender, turning eggplant several times. Cool. Peel and chop finely. In a medium bowl combine eggplant, tomato, green onions, celery, green pepper and garlic; toss to mix. Add oil, lemon juice, salt and pepper; mix well. Cover. Chill in refrigerator for 1 hour or longer to blend flavors. Makes 12 (¼-cup) servings.

Approx. per serving: 24.0 calories; 1.6 gr. fat; 60.0% calories from fat.

FRUIT KABOBS

An easy way to peel peaches is to drop them into boiling water for 30 seconds and remove. The skin should peel right away.

1 cup grapefruit juice
½ cup honey
2 tablespoons Kirsch
1 tablespoon fresh mint,
   finely chopped
3 peaches, peeled, pitted and
   halved
4 bananas, cut into 2-inch pieces
2 apples, cut into wedges
1 fresh pineapple, peeled, cored
   and cut into bite-sized pieces
2 grapefruit, sectioned
Bamboo skewers

In a small bowl combine grapefruit juice, honey, Kirsch and mint; mix well. In a shallow bowl arrange fruit. Pour grapefruit juice mixture over fruit. Marinate for 1 hour. In a shallow dish soak bamboo skewers in water to cover for 10 minutes. Preheat broiler. Drain fruit, reserving marinade. Thread fruit onto skewers. In a broiler pan place skewers. Broil for 5 minutes, brushing frequently with marinade. Makes 6 servings.

Approx. per serving: 370.0 calories; 0.9 gr. fat; 2.0% calories from fat.

STUFFED MUSHROOM CROUSTADES

These mushroom appetizers are so delicious, they just melt in your mouth. You can also use the croustade cases for other savory fillings—they're much lower in fat and calories than pastry.

**24 thin slices bread,
crusts trimmed
24 medium fresh mushrooms
1 cup fine fresh whole wheat
bread crumbs
¼ cup fresh parsley,
finely chopped
1 large clove garlic, minced
Salt and freshly ground pepper
to taste
4 teaspoons corn oil margarine
⅔ cup part-skim mozzarella
cheese, shredded**

Preheat oven to 300 degrees. With a rolling pin flatten bread. With a 1½-inch cookie cutter cut 24 rounds. Into miniature muffin cups press bread rounds. Bake for 20 to 25 minutes or until light brown. Remove from pan. Cool. Wash mushrooms and pat dry with paper towels. Remove stems and reserve for another purpose. In a food processor container combine bread crumbs, parsley, garlic and salt and pepper. Process until mixed. Add margarine. Process just until mixed. Into each mushroom cap spoon a small amount of crumb mixture. Sprinkle with cheese. Into each baked bread cup place 1 stuffed mushroom. On baking sheet arrange cups. Preheat oven to 400 degrees. Bake for 10 minutes. Broil for 1 minute if desired. Serve hot.
Makes 24 appetizers
(4 appetizers per serving).

Approx. per serving: 167.0 calories; 5.0 gr. fat; 26.94% calories from fat.

MOZZARELLA-VEGETABLE CANAPÉS

Other colorful fresh vegetables could be substituted for the carrots, radishes or green peppers.

**½ cup carrots, finely chopped
½ cup radishes, finely chopped
¼ cup onion, finely chopped
2 tablespoons green bell pepper,
finely chopped
2 tablespoons lite mayonnaise
1 tablespoons low-fat
plain yogurt
1 clove garlic, minced
½ teaspoon salt (optional)
¼ teaspoon pepper
48 small Rye Crisp crackers or
melba rounds
4 ounces part-skim mozzarella
cheese, cut into 48 small slices
Paprika**

Preheat oven to 500 degrees. In a small bowl combine carrots, radishes, onion, green pepper, mayonnaise, yogurt, garlic, salt and pepper; mix well. On each cracker spread ½ tablespoon mixture. Top with mozzarella slice and sprinkle of paprika. On baking sheet place canapés. Bake for 5 minutes. Serve immediately. Makes 48 appetizers.

Approx. per appetizer: 20.1 calories; 0.6 gr. fat; 26.86% calories from fat.

OATMEAL-SESAME STICKS

¾ cup corn oil margarine
1½ cups packed light brown sugar
1½ teaspoons vanilla extract
2¼ cups oats
¾ cup sesame seed
¾ teaspoon baking powder

Preheat oven to 375 degrees. In a large saucepan melt margarine. Add brown sugar and vanilla; blend well. Cook for 2 minutes or until bubbly; remove from heat. In a medium bowl mix oats, sesame seed and baking powder. Add to brown sugar mixture; mix well. Butter a 10 x 15-inch baking pan. Pour in batter. Bake for 7 minutes or until brown. Cool slightly. Cut into 1x2-inch bars. In the pan chill until firm. Remove from pan. In an airtight container store Oatmeal-Sesame Sticks. Makes 75 appetizers.

Approx. per appetizer: 46.0 calories; 2.6 gr. fat; 50.86% calories from fat.

CRAB-CUCUMBER ROUNDS

Crisp cucumber slices, instead of pastry or bread, make refreshing low-calorie, low-fat canapé bases.

1 Burpless cucumber
1 can (6 ounces) crab meat, drained
2 tablespoons low-fat plain yogurt
2 tablespoons chives or green onion, chopped
Salt and freshly ground pepper to taste
Paprika

With a fork score cucumber lengthwise to make a decorative edge. Slice ¼ inch thick. In a small bowl combine crab meat, yogurt, chives, salt and pepper. Place a small spoonful of crab mixture onto each cucumber slice. Sprinkle with paprika. On a serving plate arrange cucumber slices; cover with plastic wrap. Chill in refrigerator for up to 4 hours. Makes 36 appetizers.

Approx. per appetizer: 25.0 calories; 0.5 gr. fat; 18.0% calories from fat.

Photograph for this recipe on page 17.

CRAB-STUFFED CHERRY TOMATOES

Garden-fresh tomatoes are a good source of vitamin C and a colorful addition to a buffet table.

1 pint cherry tomatoes
1 can (6 ounces) crab meat
2 green onions, finely chopped
2 tablespoons dry bread crumbs
1 teaspoon fresh parsley, finely minced
1 teaspoon white wine vinegar
½ teaspoon fresh dill, finely minced or ¼ teaspoon dried dillweed
Paprika

Slice stem end from tomatoes; scoop out pulp. Invert on paper towel to drain. In a small bowl combine crab meat, green onions, bread crumbs, parsley, vinegar and dillweed; mix well. Spoon into tomatoes. Line a microwave-safe plate with paper towel. On prepared plate arrange tomatoes. Microwave on High for 2 to 4 minutes or until heated through, turning the plate several times. Sprinkle with paprika. Makes 5 servings.

Approx. per serving: 53.0 calories; 1.0 gr. fat; 16.9% calories from fat.

POLYNESIAN CRAB

The coconut in this dish gives it a sweet mysterious flavor.

1 package (6 ounces) frozen snow crab, thawed, drained and flaked
2 green onions with tops, chopped
¼ cup coconut, flaked
¼ cup lite mayonnaise
Salt and freshly ground pepper to taste
¼ teaspoon curry powder

In a medium bowl combine snow crab, green onions, coconut, mayonnaise, curry powder and salt and pepper; mix well. Refrigerate for 1 to 2 hours to blend flavors. Serve with oriental rice crackers and fresh pineapple spears. Makes 1 cup.

Approx. per serving: 26.0 calories; 1.6 gr. fat; 55.38% calories from fat.

OYSTERS ROCKEFELLER

This is an adaptation of the popular dish from New Orleans.

Rock salt
36 fresh oysters on the half shell
4 medium onions, chopped
8 ounces spinach, chopped
2 stalks celery, chopped
3 sprigs of parsley
¼ cup cream
1 teaspoon salt (optional)
¼ teaspoon black pepper
¼ teaspoon cayenne pepper

Preheat oven to 450 degrees. In 2 shallow baking dishes spread a bed of rock salt. On the bed of rock salt arrange oysters in shells. In a blender container place onions, spinach, celery, parsley, cream, salt and black and cayenne peppers. Process until puréed. Over oysters spoon purée. Bake for 4 minutes. Serve oysters on the bed of rock salt to retain heat. Makes 36 oysters.

Approx. per oyster: 25.0 calories; 0.9 gr. fat; 32.0% calories from fat.

SALMON MOUSSE WITH DILL

This smooth and creamy spread looks pretty when unmolded and surrounded with crackers, melba toast or fresh vegetables. And because it's made without whipping cream and mayonnaise, it's low in fat and calories. Be sure to use sockeye salmon for its bright red color.

½ cup water or clam juice
1 envelope unflavored gelatin
½ cup low-fat cottage cheese
1 to 2 tablespoons 1% low-fat milk
¾ cup low-fat plain yogurt
½ cup celery, finely chopped
2 tablespoons fresh dill, minced
  or 1 tablespoon dried dillweed
1 tablespoon onion, grated
1 tablespoon fresh lemon juice
1 teaspoon salt (optional)
Dash of Tabasco sauce
2 cans (7½ ounces each)
  sockeye salmon, drained

In a small saucepan pour cold water or clam juice. Sprinkle gelatin over liquid. Let stand for 5 minutes. Heat over medium heat until gelatin is dissolved. Let stand until cooled to room temperature. In a blender container combine cottage cheese and enough milk to make of desired consistency. Process until smooth. Into the gelatin mixture stir yogurt, celery, dill, onion, lemon juice, salt, Tabasco sauce and blended cottage cheese. In a bowl or food processor mash salmon with fork or process until finely flaked. Into the gelatin mixture fold salmon. Into a 4-cup mold pour salmon mixture. Cover. Chill for 3 hours or until firm. Onto a serving plate unmold mousse. Arrange crackers, melba toast or fresh vegetables around mousse. Makes 16 (¼-cup) servings.

Approx. per serving: 54.0 calories; 1.9 gr. fat; 31.66% calories from fat.

SALMON SLICES WITH LIME JUICE AND BASIL

1 pound salmon fillets with skin
½ cup fresh lime juice
2 tablespoons fresh basil or dill,
finely chopped
1 teaspoon granulated sugar
Salt and freshly ground white
pepper to taste
Fresh basil leaves

On a cutting board place fillets skin side down. With a very sharp knife slice salmon thinly; discard skin. In a shallow dish arrange salmon slices. In a small bowl combine lime juice, chopped basil, sugar and salt and pepper; mix well. Pour over salmon. Cover. Marinate in refrigerator for 5 hours. Drain, reserving marinade. On a serving platter arrange salmon slices. Over salmon drizzle a small amount of reserved marinade. Garnish with fresh basil leaves. Serve with thin slices of pumpernickel bread.
Makes 8 servings.

Approx. per serving: 86.0 calories; 3.4 gr. fat; 35.58% calories from fat.

SCALLOP CEVICHE

2 pounds fresh scallops
3 tomatoes, seeded and chopped
1 cup fresh lime juice
1 cup fresh cilantro (coriander),
chopped
1 medium onion, chopped
1 small red bell pepper, chopped
2 fresh jalapeño peppers,
seeded and minced
2 cloves garlic, minced
4 limes, cut into thin wedges
Parsley, chopped

In a colander place scallops. Rinse with cold water; drain. In a glass bowl combine scallops, tomatoes, lime juice, cilantro, onion, red and jalapeño peppers and garlic; toss gently until scallops are coated with lime juice. Cover. Marinate in refrigerator for 5 hours, stirring several times. Into individual serving bowls spoon scallop mixture. Garnish with lime wedges and parsley.
Makes 8 first-course servings.

Approx. per serving: 126.0 calories; 1.5 gr. fat; 10.71% calories from fat.

SHRIMP WRAPPED WITH SNOW PEAS

These colorful delicious hors d'oeuvres are very easy to prepare. Serve any remaining snow peas with a dip or spread, or slit them down the center and fill with cottage cheese. This dish is unusually low in fat and calories.

4 cups water
2 stalks celery with leaves
1 thick slice onion
1 clove garlic, halved
1 bay leaf
1 pound large fresh shrimp
in shells
¼ pound fresh snow peas

In a large saucepan combine 4 cups water, celery, onion slice, garlic and bay leaf. Bring to a boil; reduce heat. Simmer for 5 minutes. Add shrimp. Simmer for 3 to 5 minutes or until shrimp turn pink. Into a colander place shrimp. Drain and rinse with cold running water. Shell and devein shrimp. Trim snow peas. In a large saucepan bring several cups water to a boil. Add snow peas. Blanch for 2 minutes or just until pliable; drain. Into a bowl of ice water place shrimp to halt cooking and set color; drain. Wrap a snow pea around each shrimp; secure with a toothpick. On a serving platter arrange shrimp or insert in head of cauliflower with toothpicks. Cover. Refrigerate until serving time. Makes 4 servings.

Approx. per serving: 100.0 calories; 0.9 gr. fat; 8.1% calories from fat.

TUNA-CHEESE SOUFFLÉS

Soufflés are luscious, hot and puffy. Better volume is achieved when egg whites are beaten in a copper bowl at room temperature.

1 can (7 ounces) water-pack
white tuna or albacore, drained
¼ cup fresh parsley, chopped
¼ cup onion, chopped
2 tablespoons lite mayonnaise
6 green olives, chopped
1 tablespoon fresh lemon juice
¼ teaspoon pepper
3 egg whites
9 slices whole wheat bread
3 tablespoons Parmesan cheese,
freshly grated
3 tablespoons dry bread crumbs
Paprika to taste

Preheat oven to 250 degrees. In a blender or food processor container combine tuna, parsley, onion, mayonnaise, olives, lemon juice and pepper. Process until smooth. In a small mixer bowl beat egg whites until stiff. Fold gently into tuna mixture. Cut bread slices into fourths. On a baking sheet place bread. Bake for 30 minutes or until dry. Onto toast squares spoon tuna mixture. In a small bowl mix Parmesan cheese and bread crumbs. Sprinkle over tuna mixture. Sprinkle with paprika. Preheat broiler. Broil for 5 minutes or until light brown and bubbly. Serve immediately. Makes 36 appetizers.

Approx. per appetizer: 31.7 calories; 0.87 gr. fat; 24.7% calories from fat.

HOT MULLED APPLE CIDER

This is a wonderful alternative to hot coffee on a cool evening.

1 quart apple cider
⅔ cup packed light brown sugar
8 whole cloves
5 sticks cinnamon, divided
¼ teaspoon nutmeg
¼ teaspoon ginger
4 lemon slices

In a 1½-quart saucepan combine cider, brown sugar, cloves, 1 cinnamon stick, nutmeg and ginger. Cook over medium heat until brown sugar dissolves, stirring constantly; reduce heat. Cover. Simmer for 10 minutes. Strain. Into cups pour hot cider. Garnish with cinnamon sticks and lemon slices. May keep warm in Crock•Pot on Low.
Makes 4 (1-cup) servings.

Approx. per serving: 251.0 calories; 0.28 gr. fat; 1.0% calories from fat.

APRICOT-STRAWBERRY FRAPPÉ

1 cup apricot nectar
⅔ cup fresh orange juice
2 tablespoons honey
1 tablespoon fresh lemon juice
1 cup frozen sweetened
   strawberries, partially thawed
Mint leaves
Strawberry slices
Lemon slices

In a blender container combine apricot nectar, orange juice, honey and lemon juice. Process until mixed. Add strawberries.

Process until smooth and thickened. Into glasses pour fruit mixture. Garnish each with mint leaf, strawberry slice and lemon twist. Makes 4 servings.

Approx. per serving: 148.0 calories; 0.22 gr. fat; 0.5% calories from fat.

PEACH BELLINI

This drink became famous at Harry's American Bar in Venice. Now you can enjoy this irresistible champagne cocktail without having to travel to Italy.

2 large ripe peaches
3 tablespoons fresh orange juice
2 tablespoons fresh lemon juice
1 bottle of dry Champagne,
   chilled (optional)
1 cup small ice cubes

Into a small saucepan of boiling water drop peaches. Blanch for 2 minutes; drain. Remove peach skins and pits. In a blender container combine peaches, orange juice and lemon juice. Purée until smooth. Add Champagne and ice cubes. Process until blended and frothy. Into chilled Champagne glasses pour Champagne mixture. Serve immediately.
Makes 8 servings.

Approx. per serving: 17.38 calories; 0.05 gr. fat; 2.6% calories from fat.

BERRY-BANANA
COCKTAILS

May be poured into popsicle molds and frozen until firm.

2 cups fresh orange juice
2 bananas
1 cup fresh blueberries
½ cup fresh strawberries
½ cup fresh raspberries
2 tablespoons honey

In a blender container combine orange juice, bananas, blueberries, strawberries, raspberries and honey. Process until smooth. Into frosted glasses pour fruit mixture. Garnish with orange twists. Makes 10 servings.

Approx. per serving: 71.0 calories; 0.3 gr. fat; 4.0% calories from fat.

PAPAYA-BANANA
SMOOTHIE

2 papayas, peeled, seeded
and sliced
½ banana, peeled and sliced
4 ice cubes, crushed

In a blender or food processor place papaya and bananas. Process until smooth. Add ice cubes. Process until smooth. Into chilled glasses pour fruit mixture. Makes 4 servings.

Approx. per serving: 68.0 calories; 0.3 gr. fat; 3.97% calories from fat.

FRUIT
SLUSH

Fresh strawberries, pineapple,
peaches or other in-season fruit
Ice cubes
Club soda
Kiwifruit slices or fresh mint

In a blender container place fruit. In proportion of 2 parts ice to 1 part fruit add ice cubes 2 at a time, processing constantly. Into glass pour fruit mixture. Add enough club soda to make of desired consistency. Garnish with kiwifruit slices or fresh mint. Makes 1 serving.

Approx. per serving: 13.5 calories; 0.2 gr. fat; 13.33% calories from fat.

ICY TOMATO TUNE-UP

2½ cups tomato juice
2 tablespoons fresh lemon juice
1 teaspoon Worcestershire sauce
⅛ teaspoon celery salt
5 drops of bottled hot pepper
  sauce

In a pitcher combine tomato juice, lemon juice, Worcestershire sauce, celery salt and hot pepper sauce; mix well. Chill in refrigerator. Or pour into an 8-inch dish. Freeze until slushy. Into glasses pour or spoon tomato juice mixture. Makes 5 (4-ounce) servings.

Approx. per serving: 23.0 calories; 0.08 gr. fat; 3.0% calories from fat.

PINEAPPLE-BANANA MILK SHAKE

1 cup canned juice-pack
  crushed pineapple
1 medium banana, cut up
1 cup ice water
⅔ cup nonfat dry milk powder
2 tablespoons fresh lemon juice
¼ teaspoon vanilla extract
6 ice cubes

In a blender container combine pineapple, banana, ice water, dry milk powder, lemon juice and vanilla. Process until smooth. Add ice cubes 2 at a time, processing constantly until thick and smooth. Makes 2 servings.

Approx. per serving: 171.0 calories; 0.5 gr. fat; 2.63% calories from fat.

PINEAPPLE WASSAIL

4 cups unsweetened pineapple
  juice
2 cups fresh apple cider
1 can (12 ounces) apricot nectar
1 cup fresh orange juice
6 (1-inch) sticks cinnamon
1 teaspoon whole cloves
1 orange, sliced

In a large saucepan combine pineapple juice, cider, apricot nectar, orange juice, cinnamon sticks and cloves. Bring to a boil over medium heat; reduce heat. Simmer for 15 minutes. Into a strainer over punch bowl pour hot punch. Float orange slices in punch. Makes 9 cups.

Approx. per cup: 81.56 calories; 0.26 gr. fat; 2.9% calories from fat.

LIGHT CRANBERRY PUNCH

2 limes, sliced, divided
2 tablespoons lime juice
  concentrate
Distilled water
64 ounces cranberry juice
2 liters diet ginger ale
24 ounces white grape juice

Into a mold place half the lime slices. Add lime juice concentrate and enough distilled water to fill mold. Freeze overnight. In a punch bowl combine cranberry juice, ginger ale and grape juice. Unmold ice ring; place in punch bowl. Garnish with remaining lime slices. Makes 40 servings.

Approx. per serving: 38.0 calories; 0.1 gr. fat; 2.0% calories from fat.

HOT SPICED GRAPE PUNCH

3 tablespoons whole cloves
1 (2-inch) stick cinnamon
4 cups grape juice
½ cup water
¼ cup fresh orange juice
¼ cup fresh lemon juice

In a small cheesecloth bag tie cloves and cinnamon. In a 2-quart saucepan combine spices, grape juice and water. Bring to a boil over medium heat; remove from heat. Remove spices. Stir in orange and lemon juices. Makes 10 servings.

Approx. per serving: 42.0 calories; 0.15 gr. fat; 0.0% calories from fat.

CARD PARTY PUNCH

Make an ice ring with citrus slices for garnish to chill punch when serving from a punch bowl.

1 can (6 ounces) frozen orange
  juice concentrate, thawed
1 can (6 ounces) frozen grapefruit
  juice concentrate, thawed
2 cups diet ginger ale
2 cups water
Mint leaves

In a large pitcher combine orange juice and grapefruit juice concentrates. Add ginger ale, water and ice cubes; mix well. Into chilled glasses pour punch. Garnish with fresh mint leaves. Makes 10 (1-cup) servings.

Approx. per serving: 52.0 calories; 0.1 gr. fat; 1.7% calories from fat.

CITRUS TEA PUNCH

Herbal tea has no caffeine and makes a refreshing low-calorie punch.

1 can (6 ounces) frozen lemonade concentrate, thawed
1 can (6 ounces) frozen orange juice concentrate, thawed
2 quarts herbal or black tea, cooled
1 orange, sliced
1 lemon, sliced
6 fresh strawberries, sliced
10 to 12 fresh mint leaves

In pitchers prepare lemonade and orange juice according to package directions. In a punch bowl combine lemonade, orange juice and tea. Add orange, lemon and strawberry slices, mint leaves and ice cubes.
Makes 28 (4-ounce) servings.

Approx. per serving: 25.0 calories; 0.0 gr. fat; 0.0% calories from fat.

HOT TEA MIX

1 ¼ cups orange-flavored breakfast drink powder
¾ cup iced tea mix with lemon and sugar
1 teaspoon cinnamon
½ teaspoon allspice
½ teaspoon cloves

In a large bowl combine orange drink powder, iced tea mix, cinnamon, allspice and cloves; mix well. In an airtight container store mixture. For 1 serving combine 2 tablespoons mix and 1 cup boiling water in a cup or mug.
Makes 48 (2-tablespoon) servings.

Approx. per serving: 24.0 calories; 0.04 gr. fat; 1.5% calories from fat.

TROPICAL ICED TEA

Instead of brewing tea, try making "Sun Tea." Place 6 teabags in a ½ gallon jar and fill with 1½ quarts water. Cap loosely and place the jar in the sun for 3 to 4 hours. Remove the teabags and proceed with the recipe.

1½ quarts tea
¼ cup fresh mint leaves
Juice of 2 lemons
¼ cup pineapple juice
Granulated sugar to taste
Fresh pineapple spears

Into a pitcher pour tea. Add mint leaves. Let stand for 3 minutes. Add lemon juice, pineapple juice and sugar; mix well. Chill until serving time. Add ice cubes just before serving. Into glasses pour iced tea. Garnish with fresh pineapple spears.
Makes 12 (4-ounce) servings.

Approx. per serving: 5.4 calories; 0.0 gr. fat; 0.0% calories from fat.

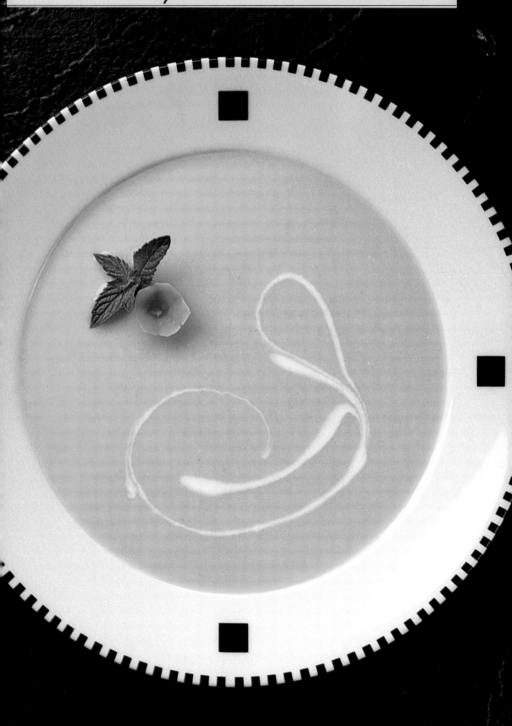

A light soup is a great way to start a meal while a hearty soup can be a meal in itself. A rich, tasty, homemade broth is the foundation for a good soup and is often an important ingredient in other dishes. If homemade broth is unavailable, there are several nutritious canned low-sodium broths on your supermarket shelves that will make very good soups or low-calorie snacks. Soups can be made from almost any food—vegetables, lentils, beans, poultry, rice—and they are low in fat and salt when you make them yourself. Avoid soups made with cream. Use vegetable purées, skim milk or buttermilk to make low-fat "cream" soups.

Fresh garden vegetables are always in abundance at your supermarket, making it easy to prepare savory salads. Choose the greenest lettuce leaves (Romaine, Boston, Bibb, Leaf) since they are highest in vitamin A. Iceberg lettuce has the least nutrition and flavor. Wash the lettuce carefully to remove any particles of sand or soil. Dry the lettuce completely. Any water that is left on the leaves prevents the dressing from clinging. After drying, store the leaves in a plastic bag in the refrigerator so they are well-chilled before serving. The dressing may be prepared hours ahead of time, but don't add it until the salad is ready to be served. Beware of regular high-fat salad dressing, bacon bits, ham, cheese and egg slices which can boost the calorie content of a salad up to 1,000 calories.

Recipe for this photograph on page 45.

BLACK BEAN SOUP

This classic Cuban soup made with frijoles negros (black beans) is a satisfying one-dish meal when served over rice and accompanied by a crisp green salad.

1 pound dried black beans, rinsed
8 cups water
1 tablespoon corn oil or safflower oil
2 medium onions, chopped
1 green pepper, chopped
1 carrot, shredded
4 cloves garlic, minced
2 teaspoons fresh oregano or 1 teaspoon dried oregano
½ teaspoon cumin seed, crushed
1 teaspoon salt (optional)
½ teaspoon pepper
2 tablespoons fresh lemon juice
2 cups hot cooked brown rice
1 cup low-fat plain yogurt
Chopped green onions

In a large saucepan soak beans in water overnight or bring to the boiling point over medium-high heat, boil for 2 minutes, remove from heat, cover and let stand for 1 hour. In a skillet heat oil over medium heat. Add onions, green pepper, carrot, garlic, oregano and cumin. Sauté until vegetables are soft. Stir into beans. Add salt and pepper. Bring to a boil; reduce heat. Cover. Simmer for 1½ to 2 hours or until beans are very tender, stirring occasionally. Stir in lemon juice. Into soup bowls spoon rice. Ladle bean soup over rice. Top with yogurt and green onions. Makes 8 servings.

Approx. per serving: 314.0 calories; 5.5 gr. fat; 15.76% calories from fat.

BEAN AND BASIL SOUP

Hearty with beans, garlic and potato, this soup goes well before a main course. It can also be served as a main course in itself accompanied by a basket of crusty breads, a crisp salad and fresh fruit.

3 quarts water
3 cups onions, diced
2 cups carrots, diced
1 cup potato, diced
1 teaspoon salt (optional)
2 cups fresh green beans or 2 packages (10 ounces each) frozen green beans
1 cup uncooked macaroni
¼ cup tomato paste
¼ cup Parmesan cheese, freshly grated
2 tablespoons fresh basil or 2 teaspoons dried basil
3 cloves garlic, mashed
1 can (16 ounces) white beans, drained

In a stockpot combine water, onions, carrots, potato and salt. Cook over medium heat until vegetables are almost tender. Add green beans and macaroni. Cook until vegetables and macaroni are tender. In a small bowl combine tomato paste, cheese, basil and garlic; mix well. Stir 2 cups hot soup vigorously into cheese mixture; stir cheese mixture into hot soup. Add beans. Cook until heated through. Makes 6 servings.

Approx. per serving: 306.0 calories; 4.7 gr. fat; 13.82% calories from fat; high vitamin A; high fiber.

IT'S ALMOST SOUP

8 cups water
2 cups Bean 'N' Grain Mix
1 large onion, chopped
1 tablespoon fresh lemon juice
1 tablespoon honey
1 clove garlic, minced
1 bay leaf
Salt and pepper to taste
1 can (24 ounces) vegetable juice
1 can (16 ounces) tomatoes
2 cups fresh carrots, sliced
1 ½ cups cabbage, shredded
1 cup celery, chopped

In a 5-quart stockpot combine 8 cups water and 2 cups bean mix. Bring to a boil over medium-high heat; reduce heat. Cover. Simmer for 2 minutes; remove from heat. Let stand, covered, for 1 hour. Do not drain. Add onion, lemon juice, honey, garlic, bay leaf and salt and pepper. Cover. Simmer for 2 hours. Add vegetable juice, tomatoes with liquid, carrots, cabbage and celery. Cover. Simmer for 30 minutes or until vegetables are tender. Discard bay leaf. Makes 6 to 8 servings.

Approx. per serving: 330.0 calories; 1.6 gr. fat; 4.36% calories from fat; high vitamin A; high fiber.

Bean 'N' Grain Mix
1 pound dried lima beans
1 pound dried pinto beans
1 pound dried kidney beans
1 pound dried navy beans
1 pound dried garbanzo beans (chick peas)
1 pound dried lentils
1 pound dried black-eyed peas
1 pound dried yellow or green split peas
1 pound dried Great Northern beans
1 pound dried butter beans
1 pound dried fava beans
1 pound pearl barley
1 pound brown rice

In a large container combine 7 or more of the dried ingredients; mix well. In 2-cup containers or plastic bags package the mixture. Use some as gifts, adding a copy of the soup recipe to each package. Makes 7 to 13 pounds.

WHITE BEAN AND SPINACH SOUP

1 pound dried white beans
8 cups water, divided
8 cups beef broth, either homemade or canned
2 cups fresh carrots, grated
1 ½ cups onions, chopped
4 cloves garlic, minced
1 teaspoon fresh thyme or ½ teaspoon dried thyme
3 bay leaves
¼ teaspoon black pepper
⅛ teaspoon cayenne pepper
6 cups fresh spinach, torn
2 cans (16 ounces each) tomatoes, coarsely chopped
½ teaspoon granulated sugar
½ teaspoon salt (omit if using canned broth)

In a large saucepan soak beans in 4 cups water overnight. Drain soaking water. Add beef broth and 4 cups fresh water. Bring to a boil over medium-high heat; reduce heat. Add carrots, onions, garlic, thyme, bay leaves and black and cayenne peppers. Bring to a boil; reduce heat. Cover. Simmer for 1 hour or until beans are tender. Add spinach, tomatoes with liquid, sugar and salt. Bring to a boil; reduce heat. Simmer for 5 minutes. Discard bay leaves. Makes 8 servings.

Approx. per serving: 240.0 calories; 1.8 gr. fat; 6.75% calories from fat; high vitamin A; high fiber.

CHILLED SPINACH BORSCHT

This light and elegant soup is the perfect start to a meal. And best of all, it can be thrown together in practically no time at all. Be sure to wash the spinach thoroughly to release any sand.

1 pound fresh spinach or
1 package (10 ounces) frozen spinach, thawed
1 large cucumber, peeled and chopped
½ medium yellow onion, chopped
1 cup skim-milk buttermilk, divided
4 cups chicken stock, either homemade or canned
1 teaspoon vinegar
½ teaspoon fresh dill, chopped or ¼ teaspoon dried dillweed
Salt and pepper to taste
Chopped cucumber

Rinse spinach well. In a saucepan place spinach and a small amount of salted water. Cook over medium heat until tender. Drain and chop. Into a blender container place cucumber and onion. Process until puréed. Into a large bowl place purée. Stir in half the buttermilk. Add chicken stock and vinegar; blend well. Stir in spinach, remaining buttermilk, dill and salt and pepper. Chill until serving time. Into soup bowls ladle soup. Garnish with chopped cucumber. Makes 8 to 10 servings.

Approx. per serving: 53.0 calories; 1.3 gr. fat; 22.07% calories from fat.

VEGETABLE BORSCHT

Serve small portions of this colorful, bursting-with-flavor soup for a first course, or larger servings for a main course. Leftover soup may be frozen.

4 cups beef or chicken stock, either homemade or canned
2 large fresh beets, peeled and chopped
1 large potato, peeled and chopped
1 onion, chopped
1 medium carrot, sliced
¼ small head cabbage, shredded
1 tomato, chopped
2 tablespoons fresh parsley, chopped or 1 tablespoon dried parsley
1 teaspoon fresh dill, chopped or ½ teaspoon dried dillweed
1 teaspoon fresh lemon juice
1 teaspoon salt (optional)
Freshly ground pepper to taste
3 tablespoons low-fat plain yogurt or Mock Sour Cream (see page 84)

In a large saucepan combine stock, beets, potato, onion and carrot. Bring to a boil over medium-high heat; reduce heat. Cover. Simmer for 30 minutes. Skim if necessary. Add cabbage, tomato, parsley and dill. Cover. Simmer for 30 minutes longer or until vegetables are tender. Add lemon juice, salt and pepper. Into soup bowls ladle soup. Garnish each serving with 1 rounded teaspoon yogurt or Mock Sour Cream. Makes 8 servings.

Approx. per serving: 64.5 calories; 1.0 gr. fat; 13.95% calories from fat.

CABBAGE SOUP

Soup is even more appetizing when it is garnished with a flourish at the moment of serving. So, add a sprinkling of freshly chopped herbs or freshly ground black pepper to zip up this savory soup.

4 cups water
4 cups cabbage, grated
3 cups potatoes, unpeeled, diced
2 cups carrots, chopped
1 cup onion, chopped
1 cup celery with leaves, chopped
1 teaspoon fresh thyme or
  ½ teaspoon dried thyme
1 bay leaf
½ teaspoon salt (optional)
¼ teaspoon pepper
2 cups 1% low-fat milk
1 can (15 ounces) tomato sauce

In a large saucepan over medium-high heat bring water to a boil. Add cabbage, potatoes, carrots, onion, celery, thyme, bay leaf, salt and pepper. Bring to a boil; reduce heat. Simmer, uncovered, for 45 minutes or until vegetables are tender. Add milk and tomato sauce. Heat over low heat to serving temperature. Remove and discard bay leaf.
Makes 8 servings.

Approx. per serving: 119.0 calories; 1.0 gr. fat; 7.56% calories from fat; high vitamin A.

HOMEMADE CHICKEN BROTH

You can make stock whenever you have the ingredients on hand and freeze it in small containers to use when needed.

1 (2-pound) stewing chicken,
  skin and fat removed
3 quarts water
2 carrots, peeled and quartered
2 stalks celery, coarsely chopped
1 onion, quartered
2 sprigs of fresh parsley
8 peppercorns
1 bay leaf

In a large stockpot combine chicken, water, carrots, celery, onion, parsley, peppercorns and bay leaf. Bring to a boil over medium-high heat, skimming as necessary. Reduce heat when no more foam rises to the top. Simmer, uncovered, for 1 to 2 hours. Strain broth. Refrigerate until any fat rises to the top and congeals. Remove and discard fat.
Makes 12 cups.

Approx. per serving: 114.0 calories; 1.0 gr. fat; 7.0% calories from fat.

HOMEMADE VEGETABLE BROTH

This broth can be used as a base for other soups.

1 gallon water
4 tomatoes, seeded and coarsely
  chopped
4 celery stalks, thickly sliced
3 carrots, peeled and
  thickly sliced
2 onions, cut into wedges
2 leeks, white part only, washed
  and thickly sliced
2 turnips, peeled and
  cut into wedges
1 red or green bell pepper,
  stemmed, seeded and
  cut into chunks
1 zucchini, ends trimmed and
  thickly sliced
3 cloves garlic
2 sprigs of Italian parsley
1 tablespoon fresh thyme or
  1 ½ teaspoons dried thyme
2 bay leaves
10 black peppercorns

In a large stockpot combine water, tomatoes, celery, carrots, onions, leeks, turnips, bell pepper and zucchini. Add garlic, parsley, thyme, bay leaves and peppercorns. Bring to a boil over medium-high heat; reduce heat. Simmer, uncovered, for 2 hours. Strain and discard solids. Cool to room temperature. Makes 16 cups.

Approx. per serving: 14.0 calories; 0.06 gr. fat; 3.0% calories from fat.

CREAM OF BROCCOLI SOUP

Our favorite broccoli soup tastes purely and simply of broccoli. It's wonderful hot, but it's also fabulous chilled. Make enough and you can have it both ways. Cauliflower may be substituted for broccoli.

3 cups broccoli florets and
  peeled stems, finely chopped
1 ½ cups water
1 tablespoon corn oil margarine
½ cup onion, chopped
1 tablespoon all-purpose flour
3 cups 1% low-fat milk
½ teaspoon salt (optional)
½ teaspoon black pepper
¼ teaspoon paprika
¼ teaspoon celery seed
⅛ teaspoon cayenne pepper

In a 3-quart saucepan combine broccoli and water. Bring to a boil over medium-high heat; reduce heat. Cover. Simmer for 10 minutes. Drain, reserving liquid. In a larger saucepan over low heat melt margarine. Add onion. Sauté until soft. Add flour. Cook for several seconds, stirring constantly. Stir in reserved liquid. Cook until thickened, stirring constantly. Add milk, broccoli, salt, black pepper, paprika, celery seed and cayenne pepper; mix well. Heat to serving temperature over low heat. Makes 6 servings.

Approx. per serving: 101.0 calories; 3.32 gr. fat; 29.58% calories from fat; high fiber.

CHICKEN AND BEAN TUREEN

2 chicken legs
2 chicken breasts
2 onions, chopped, divided
5 carrots, divided
1 stalk celery
2 cans (15 ounces each)
 Great Northern beans,
 drained and rinsed
2 tomatoes, peeled and chopped
½ green bell pepper, chopped
2 teaspoons fresh thyme or
 1 teaspoon dried thyme
2 cloves garlic, minced
Parsley to taste
Salt and pepper to taste

Remove all skin and fat from chicken pieces. In a saucepan place chicken, half of the onion, 1 sliced carrot and celery. Add water to cover. Cook over medium heat until chicken is tender. Cool. Bone chicken. Strain and reserve 2 cups broth. Preheat oven to 350 degrees. Grease a large casserole. In the prepared casserole place chicken, reserved broth and beans. Cut the remaining 4 carrots into large pieces. Add carrots with tomatoes, remaining onion, green pepper, thyme, garlic, parsley and salt and pepper. Bake for 45 minutes or until mixture simmers gently. Serve in soup bowls.
Makes 6 servings.

Approx. per serving: 354.0 calories; 6.6 gr. fat; 16.77% calories from fat; very high vitamin A; high fiber.

CHICKEN-CABBAGE SOUP

3 cups chicken broth, either
 homemade or canned
3 cups water
2 cups fresh tomatoes, chopped
1 potato, peeled and chopped
½ cup carrot, shredded
½ cup celery, chopped
½ cup onion, chopped
4 peppercorns
1 bay leaf
3 cups cabbage, shredded
1 cup cooked boneless, skinless
 chicken, chopped
¼ cup fresh lemon juice
1 tablespoon granulated sugar

In a large saucepan combine broth, water, tomatoes, potato, carrot, celery and onion. Add peppercorns and bay leaf. Simmer for 1 hour, stirring occasionally. Add cabbage. Simmer for 10 minutes. Add chicken, lemon juice and sugar. Heat to serving temperature. Remove bay leaf.
Makes 6 to 8 servings.

Approx. per serving: 113.0 calories; 2.3 gr. fat; 18.31% calories from fat.

CHINESE CHICKEN-NOODLE SOUP

This is a very simple soup that can make use of leftover chicken or turkey. The ginger, soy sauce and Sherry seasonings give the soup a Chinese accent. Vermicelli is added as a delicious fillip.

8 cups chicken broth, either homemade or canned
½ pound chicken or turkey breast, skinned, boned and cut into small pieces
4 scallions, sliced
3 carrots, sliced
2 tablespoons lite soy sauce
1 tablespoon granulated sugar
1 tablespoon Sherry
½ teaspoon fresh gingerroot, finely minced
4 ounces whole wheat vermicelli, broken into 1-inch pieces

In a large soup pot place chicken broth. Bring to a boil over medium-high heat. Add chicken, scallions, carrots, soy sauce, sugar, Sherry and ginger; reduce heat. Cover. Simmer for 20 minutes. Bring to a boil; add vermicelli. Cook over medium-high heat for 15 minutes. Skim. Into soup bowls ladle soup. Makes 8 servings.

Approx. per serving: 136.0 calories; 2.17 gr. fat; 14.36% calories from fat; high vitamin A.

CHICKEN GUMBO

1 pound boneless skinless chicken breast, cut into bite-sized pieces
3 cups water
2 cups chicken broth, either homemade or canned, divided
1 cup onion, chopped
1 clove garlic, minced
½ teaspoon fresh thyme or ¼ teaspoon dried thyme
¼ teaspoon dried red peppers
¼ teaspoon fresh sage or ⅛ teaspoon dried sage
1 bay leaf
2 cups fresh okra, sliced
2 cups fresh tomatoes, chopped
2 cups fresh corn
½ teaspoon salt (optional)
¼ teaspoon pepper
2 cups uncooked brown rice
1 tablespoon corn oil margarine
1 tablespoon all-purpose flour

Rinse chicken. In a large soup pot place chicken, water and 1 cup broth. Bring to a boil over medium-high heat; reduce heat. Skim with slotted spoon. Add onion, garlic, thyme, red peppers, sage and bay leaf. Cover. Simmer for 20 minutes. Skim. Add okra, tomatoes and corn. Cover. Simmer for 20 minutes. Add salt and pepper. Cook rice according to package directions. In a medium saucepan over low heat melt margarine. Add flour. Cook until golden and bubbly, stirring constantly. Stir in 1 cup broth. Bring to a boil, stirring constantly; reduce heat. Whisk until smooth. Stir into chicken mixture. Heat to serving temperature. Into large soup bowls spoon hot cooked brown rice. Ladle gumbo over rice. Makes 8 servings.

Approx. per serving: 317.0 calories; 4.9 gr. fat; 13.91% calories from fat; high fiber.

NEW ENGLAND SEAFOOD CHOWDER

Enjoy the freshest catch of the day, transformed into a soup of the sea. Choose from grouper, red snapper, yellowtail or flounder. Just cooking the fish a few minutes produces a broth rich in body and flavor.

4 slices whole wheat bread
2 tablespoons corn oil margarine
4 cups onions, sliced
2 tablespoons all-purpose flour
2 cups clam juice
2 cups water
5 cups potatoes, sliced
2 teaspoons fresh thyme or
 1 teaspoon dried thyme
¾ teaspoon salt (optional)
½ teaspoon pepper
2 pounds boneless fish fillets,
 cut into bite-sized pieces
2 cups 1% low-fat milk
½ cup fresh parsley, chopped

Preheat oven to 250 degrees. Cut bread into cubes. On a baking sheet spread cubes in a single layer. Bake for 30 minutes or until dry. Croutons should measure about 1½ cups. In a soup pot over low heat melt margarine. Add onions. Sauté for 10 minutes. Stir in flour. Cook for 2 minutes, stirring constantly. Add clam juice and water. Bring to a boil over medium-high heat, stirring constantly. Add potatoes, thyme, salt and pepper; reduce heat. Simmer for 10 minutes. Add fish and milk. Simmer for 5 minutes or just until fish is opaque; do not overcook. Into soup bowls ladle soup. Sprinkle with parsley and croutons. Makes 12 first-course or 8 main-dish servings.

Approx. per serving: 198.0 calories; 4.96 gr. fat; 22.54% calories from fat.

CURRIED WINTER SQUASH SOUP

Winter squash and crisp apples make this soup a special starter for any occasion. It is easy to make ahead and ideal to have on hand for spur-of-the-moment entertaining.

Corn oil
1½ cups onions, finely chopped
4 to 5 teaspoons curry powder
2 medium (2½ pounds) butternut
 squash
3 cups low-sodium chicken broth,
 either homemade or canned
1 medium apple, peeled, cored
 and chopped
1 cup apple juice
Salt and freshly ground pepper
 to taste

In a large saucepan over low heat melt margarine. Add onions and curry powder. Cover. Simmer for 20 minutes or until onions are soft. Peel, seed and chop squash. Add squash, broth and apple to saucepan. Bring to a boil over medium-high heat; reduce heat. Cover partially. Simmer for 25 minutes or until squash and apple are very tender. Strain; reserve liquid and solids. In a food processor fitted with a steel blade or in a blender process solids until smooth. Add 1 cup reserved liquid. Process until smooth. To the saucepan return the puréed soup. Add enough remaining reserved soup liquid and apple juice to make of desired consistency. Add salt and pepper. Heat to serving temperature. Serve immediately. May substitute pumpkin or other winter squash for butternut. Substitute 1% low-fat milk for apple juice for a less sweet taste. Makes 8 servings.

Approx. per serving: 100.0 calories; 2.8 gr. fat; 25.2% calories from fat; high vitamin A.

CURRIED CARROT SOUP

Although particularly appropriate for the holidays, this favorite soup is good and easy to prepare year round. Sautéing the spices brings out their flavor.

1 tablespoon corn oil margarine
4 cups carrots, chopped
1 cup onion, chopped
½ teaspoon curry powder
½ teaspoon cumin
½ teaspoon coriander
5 cups water
½ teaspoon salt (optional)
¼ teaspoon white pepper
1 cup low-fat cottage cheese
1 cup 1% low-fat milk
1 teaspoon fresh lemon juice
½ cup green bell pepper, chopped
½ cup fresh parsley, chopped

In a large soup pot over low heat melt margarine. Add carrots and onion. Sauté for 5 minutes, adding curry powder, cumin and coriander. Add water, salt and white pepper. Bring to a boil over medium-high heat; reduce heat. Cover partially. Simmer for 15 minutes. Into a blender container pour carrot mixture. Process until puréed. Return to the soup pot. In the blender container place cottage cheese, milk and lemon juice. Process until smooth. Pour into carrot mixture. Heat to serving temperature over low heat. Into soup bowls ladle soup. Garnish with green pepper and parsley. Soup may be served chilled.
Makes 6 servings.

Approx. per serving: 111.0 calories; 3.73 gr. fat; 30.24% calories from fat; very high vitamin A.

Photograph for this recipe on page 35.

GAZPACHO SOUP

This enormously popular cold summer soup is really a liquid salad. It originated in Andalucia, Spain, but it is now enjoyed in all corners of the world. It is customary to serve the gazpacho and then pass small bowls containing croutons, onion, cucumber, green pepper and tomato for the diner to sprinkle on top.

6 large ripe tomatoes, seeded
    and chopped or 1 ½ cups
    canned imported plum
    tomatoes, drained
2 red bell peppers, cored, seeded
    and coarsely chopped
2 large cucumbers, peeled,
    seeded and coarsely chopped
1 medium yellow onion, coarsely
    chopped
1 clove garlic
1 ½ cups canned tomato juice
¼ cup red wine vinegar
1 tablespoon olive oil
Pinch of cayenne pepper or
    dash of Tabasco sauce
Salt and freshly ground
    black pepper to taste
½ cup fresh parsley, chopped

In a food processor fitted with a metal blade or in a blender container place tomatoes, red peppers, cucumbers, onion and garlic a small amount at a time, adding enough tomato juice to each batch to keep blades from clogging. Process until well mixed; do not purée completely. In a large bowl combine processed vegetable mixture, vinegar, olive oil, cayenne pepper and salt and black pepper. Cover. Refrigerate for 4 hours or longer. Adjust seasonings if necessary. Into soup bowls ladle soup. Garnish with parsley.
Makes 8 servings.

Approx. per serving: 64.0 calories; 2.2 gr. fat; 30.93% calories from fat; high fiber.

FRENCH ONION SOUP

This soup warmed the hearts and stomachs of truckers at the old Les Halles Market in Paris. Although the market no longer exists, the memories of this heady combination of onions and broth topped with golden slices of cheese-laden toast linger on. You can make it easily in your own kitchen filling the house with irresistible aromas.

2 tablespoons corn oil margarine
1 ½ pounds onions, quartered and thinly sliced
2 cups fresh carrots, grated
1 tablespoon light brown sugar
3 tablespoons all-purpose flour
1 teaspoon paprika
6 cups beef broth, either homemade or canned
1 teaspoon fresh thyme or ½ teaspoon dried thyme
¼ teaspoon salt (omit if using canned broth)
¼ teaspoon pepper
6 slices (1 to 1 ½ ounces each) whole wheat or white French bread
⅓ cup part-skim mozzarella cheese, grated

In a large soup pot over low heat melt margarine. Add onions and carrots. Cover. Cook over very low heat for 20 minutes. Add brown sugar. Cook until onions are brown, stirring constantly. Add flour and paprika; stir until onions are coated. Add broth, thyme, salt and pepper; mix well. Bring to a boil over medium-high heat, stirring constantly; reduce heat. Simmer, uncovered, for 30 minutes. Preheat oven to 250 degrees. On a baking sheet place bread. In oven dry bread slices for 30 minutes to make croutons. Into ovenproof soup bowls ladle soup. Onto a baking sheet place the soup bowls. Into each bowl place 1 crouton; sprinkle with cheese. Place 4 inches below broiler. Broil for 3 to 4 minutes or until cheese is lightly browned and bubbly. If your soup bowls are not oven-proof, place cheese-topped croutons on baking sheet; broil until bubbly. Into soup bowls ladle piping hot soup and top with croutons. Makes 6 servings.

Approx. per serving: 233.0 calories; 5.5 gr. fat; 21.24% calories from fat; high vitamin A.

CHILLED MELON AND YOGURT SOUP

A hint of ginger and fresh mint heightens the flavor of this light, refreshing summer soup. Serve it as a first course for brunch, lunch or dinner. Be sure the cantaloupe you use is ripe.

1 ripe cantaloupe
1 cup low-fat plain yogurt
3 tablespoons fresh lemon juice
½ teaspoon fresh gingerroot, peeled and grated or ¼ teaspoon dried ginger
2 tablespoons fresh mint leaves, chopped

Cut cantaloupe into halves; discard seed. Into a food processor or blender container scoop cantaloupe pulp. Process until puréed. Yield should be about 1 ½ cups. Add yogurt, lemon juice and ginger. Process until blended. Refrigerate until serving time. Into small bowls pour cantaloupe mixture. Garnish with fresh mint. Makes 4 servings.

Approx. per serving: 95.8 calories; 1.32 gr. fat; 12.4% calories from fat; high vitamin A.

LEEK AND POTATO SOUP

The base for this delicious soup freezes well; just thaw, add milk and serve hot or cold for a first course at a dinner party. For a lunch main course, top soup with garlic croutons, baby shrimp and chopped chives or green onions.

6 medium leeks
8 cups chicken stock, either
  homemade or canned
4 medium potatoes, peeled and
  chopped
1 clove garlic, minced
1 cup 1% low-fat milk
Salt and freshly ground pepper
  to taste
3 tablespoons fresh parsley or
  chives, minced

Trim leeks, leaving about 2 inches of green portion. Cut lengthwise halfway through white portion. Spread leeks apart; rinse well under cold running water. Slice thinly by hand or in food processor. In a large saucepan combine leeks, chicken stock, potatoes and garlic. Bring to a boil over medium-high heat; reduce heat. Cover partially. Simmer for 30 minutes or until vegetables are tender. In a blender or food processor purée vegetable mixture. Into a saucepan pour purée. Heat to serving temperature over low heat. Stir in milk and salt and pepper. Into soup cups ladle soup. Garnish with parsley. Soup may be cooled, poured into freezer containers and frozen after puréeing. Makes 12 cups.

Approx. per cup: 94.0 calories; 1.3 gr. fat; 12.44 % calories from fat.

LENTIL SOUP

This thick, zesty soup with its hint of vinegar is lovely on cool evenings.

1 tablespoon olive oil
2 cups dried lentils
1 cup onion, chopped
1 cup fresh carrots, chopped
¼ cup fresh parsley, chopped
2 cloves garlic, minced
¾ teaspoon salt (optional)
½ teaspoon pepper
1 teaspoon fresh thyme or
  ½ teaspoon dried thyme
8 cups water
2 cups fresh tomatoes, chopped
2 tablespoons white or red wine
  vinegar

In a soup pot heat olive oil over medium heat. Add lentils, onion, carrots, parsley, garlic, salt, pepper and thyme. Sauté over medium heat for 15 minutes. Add water and tomatoes. Cover; reduce heat. Simmer for 1½ hours. Add vinegar. Simmer for 30 minutes longer. Makes 10 servings.

Approx. per serving: 170.0 calories; 1.5 gr. fat; 7.94% calories from fat; high fiber.

THICK AND HEARTY MINESTRONE

Nothing is better on a winter evening than a bowl of thick, hearty, steaming vegetable soup. Although thick with vegetables, this Italian specialty is not heavy and can precede a pasta course. It's also good for a soup-and-sandwich meal.

3 tablespoons olive oil
1 large onion, chopped
6 large fresh mushrooms, sliced
3 cloves garlic, chopped
1 tablespoon fresh basil or
   1 ½ teaspoons dried basil
1 teaspoon fresh oregano or
   ½ teaspoon dried oregano
1 teaspoon fresh parsley
5 cups water
1 can (20 ounces) mixed
   vegetable juice cocktail
4 carrots, thinly sliced
2 zucchini, sliced
½ small head cabbage, shredded
½ cup elbow macaroni

In a 6-quart saucepan heat olive oil over medium heat. Add onion, mushrooms, garlic, basil, oregano and parsley. Sauté for several minutes. Add water and vegetable juice cocktail. Bring to a boil over medium-high heat. Add carrots, zucchini, cabbage and macaroni. Cook just until vegetables and macaroni are tender. Makes 8 servings.

Approx. per serving: 98.0 calories; 2.0 gr. fat; 18.36% calories from fat; high vitamin A; high fiber.

ORIENTAL SPINACH SOUP

1 package (10 ounces) frozen
   chopped spinach
1 tablespoon cornstarch
1 ½ cups water, divided
2 cans (10 ½ ounces each)
   chicken broth
½ cup celery, diagonally sliced
½ cup fresh carrots, thinly sliced
2 tablespoons green onions, sliced
2 teaspoons lite soy sauce

Cook spinach according to package directions, omitting salt; drain well. In a saucepan dissolve cornstarch in ¼ cup water. Stir in remaining 1¼ cups water and chicken broth. Add spinach, celery, carrots, green onions and soy sauce. Bring to a boil over medium-high heat, stirring constantly. Cook until clear and thickened, stirring constantly. Reduce heat. Simmer for 5 minutes. Makes 8 cups (1⅓ cups per serving).

Approx. per serving: 30.6 calories; 0.5 gr. fat; 14.7% calories from fat; high vitamin A.

SMART STEWP

This soup that's almost a stew thickens and improves with flavor as it mellows overnight in the refrigerator.

4¼ cups water, divided
1 medium onion, chopped
1 can (46 ounces) tomato juice
1 package (16 ounces) frozen mixed vegetables
1 can (14½ ounces) tomatoes
2 cups celery, chopped
1 cup Napa or green cabbage, shredded
1 cup uncooked brown rice
¼ cup fresh parsley, chopped
2 teaspoons fresh oregano or 1 teaspoon dried oregano
1 teaspoon celery seed
1 teaspoon dillseed
1 teaspoon chives, chopped
Spice Blend seasoning to taste (see page 78)

In a nonstick skillet heat ¼ cup water over low heat. Add onion. Simmer until onion is clear. Into a soup pot place onion. Add the remaining 4 cups water, tomato juice, mixed vegetables, tomatoes, celery, cabbage, rice, parsley, oregano, celery seed, dillseed, chives and Spice Blend. Bring to a boil over medium-high heat; reduce heat. Simmer for 30 minutes or until rice is tender. Refrigerate overnight. Reheat to serving temperature over low heat.
Makes 3 quarts.

Approx. per serving: 112.0 calories; 0.74 gr. fat; 5.94% calories from fat; high fiber.

SPLIT PEA AND BARLEY SOUP

This hearty soup could be served as a first course for any kind of meal, formal or informal. It is also good for a soup-and-sandwich meal.

6 cups chicken broth, either homemade or canned
1½ cups dried split peas
½ medium onion, coarsely chopped
½ carrot, coarsely chopped
1 stalk celery, coarsely chopped
1 clove garlic, minced
½ cup pearl barley
Salt and freshly ground white pepper to taste

In a 3-quart soup pot place broth, split peas, onion, carrot, celery and garlic. Bring to a boil over medium-high heat; reduce heat. Simmer, uncovered, for 1 hour. In a food processor or blender container process soup a small amount at a time. In a soup pot combine puréed soup and barley. Bring to a boil; reduce heat. Simmer for 30 to 40 minutes or until barley is tender. Add salt and white pepper. Makes 6 servings.

Approx. per serving: 265.0 calories; 1.9 gr. fat; 6.45% calories from fat.

CHILLED FRESH TOMATO SOUP

This is a delicious and easy way to use an abundance of fresh tomatoes. Dishes of chopped scallions, cucumber and zucchini may be served as garnishes.

4 pounds fresh tomatoes
2 cups chicken broth, either
 homemade or canned
2 tablespoons onion, chopped
2 teaspoons granulated sugar
½ teaspoon fresh basil or
 ¼ teaspoon dried basil
½ teaspoon salt (optional)
¼ teaspoon pepper

Into a large saucepan of boiling water dip tomatoes for 30 seconds. Into a large bowl of cold water place tomatoes immediately. Let stand until cool enough to handle. Peel with knife; skin should slip off easily. Cut each tomato in half crosswise; squeeze gently to remove seed. Cut core from tomato; cut into quarters. In a blender container place ¼ of the tomatoes at a time. Process until puréed. In a large bowl combine tomatoes, chicken broth, onion, sugar, basil, salt and pepper. Refrigerate for several hours to blend flavors. Serve chilled.
Makes 6 servings.

Approx. per serving: 92.4 calories; 1.0 gr. fat; 9.74% calories from fat; high fiber.

TOMATO BOUILLON

3 cans (1 pound each) tomatoes
1 cup turnips, chopped
1 cup onion, chopped
2 carrots, chopped
½ green bell pepper, chopped
1 teaspoon fresh thyme or
 ½ teaspoon dried thyme
½ teaspoon granulated sugar
¼ teaspoon salt (optional)
4 peppercorns
¼ cup Port
1 tablespoon fresh lemon juice
6 tablespoons fresh parsley,
 chopped

In a soup pot place tomatoes with liquid; break apart with fork. Add turnips, onion, carrots, green pepper, thyme, sugar, salt and peppercorns. Cover tightly. Bring to a boil over medium-high heat; reduce heat. Simmer for 1 hour, stirring 1 or 2 times. Cool. Into a sieve pour hot vegetable mixture. Press through sieve into a saucepan. Add wine and lemon juice. Bring to a boil; reduce heat. Simmer for 5 minutes. Into soup bowls, ladle soup. Garnish each serving with 1 tablespoon parsley. Makes 6 servings.

Approx. per serving: 83.0 calories; 0.7 gr. fat; 5.31% calories from fat; high vitamin A.

TOMATO-ZUCCHINI SOUP

Fresh cilantro is a pungent and aromatic herb used extensively in Asian cooking. It is sometimes called coriander or Chinese parsley. Coriander seeds are the fruit of the plant and taste nothing like fresh cilantro (coriander). Cilantro and tomatoes make a perfect marriage in this piquant soup.

1 tablespoon corn oil margarine
½ cup celery, chopped
3 shallots, chopped
2 large cloves garlic, minced
4 cups chicken stock, either homemade or canned
3 tomatoes, chopped
1 zucchini, thinly sliced
1 tablespoon tomato paste
1 teaspoon fresh parsley, chopped or ½ teaspoon dried parsley
½ teaspoon fresh cilantro (coriander)
1 bay leaf
4 to 6 tablespoons low-fat plain yogurt

In a soup pot over low heat melt margarine. Add celery, shallots and garlic. Sauté until tender. Add chicken stock, tomatoes, zucchini, tomato paste, parsley, cilantro and bay leaf. Simmer for 2 hours. Discard bay leaf. Into soup bowls ladle soup. Garnish with yogurt. Makes 4 to 6 servings.

Approx. per serving: 115.0 calories; 3.75 gr. fat; 29.34% calories from fat.

VEGETABLE SOUP WITH PASTA

1 tablespoon olive oil
2 cups onions, chopped
1 pound fresh carrots, sliced
1 large green or red bell pepper, chopped
2 cloves garlic, minced
10 cups chicken broth, either homemade or canned
2 cups unpeeled potatoes, chopped
2 cups turnips, chopped
2 pounds fresh green beans, sliced
2 cups cooked tri-colored small pasta shells
½ teaspoon salt (optional)
¼ teaspoon pepper
1½ cups parsley, chopped

In a soup pot heat olive oil over medium heat. Add onions. Sauté until tender. Add carrots, bell pepper and garlic. Cook for 5 minutes. Add chicken broth, potatoes and turnips. Bring to a boil; reduce heat. Cover partially. Cook for 10 minutes or until potatoes and turnips are almost tender. Add green beans. Simmer for 5 minutes. Add pasta, salt and pepper. Simmer for 10 minutes longer. Into soup bowls ladle soup. Garnish each with 2 tablespoons parsley. Makes 12 servings.

Approx. per serving: 152.0 calories; 2.9 gr. fat; 17.17% calories from fat; high vitamin A; high fiber.

ICED SUMMER FRUIT SALAD

1 medium cantaloupe
½ medium honeydew melon
1 papaya
1 pound seedless grapes

Peel and seed cantaloupe and honeydew; cut into bite-sized pieces. Peel papaya and cut into bite-sized pieces. In a large bowl place melon pieces, papaya pieces and grapes. Add dressing; toss gently. Chill until serving time. May cut melons and papaya into slices. On a large platter arrange overlapping slices. Sprinkle grapes over slices. Drizzle a small amount of dressing over fruit. Into a small serving bowl pour remaining dressing. Makes 8 servings.

Dressing
½ cup plain low-fat yogurt
2 tablespoons apricot preserves
2 tablespoons fresh orange juice

In a small bowl combine yogurt, preserves and orange juice; blend well.

Approx. per serving: 111.0 calories; 0.82 gr. fat; 6.64% calories from fat.

SUMMER FRUIT SALAD WITH MOZZARELLA CHEESE

This combination of fresh seasonal fruits can begin or end a meal on a very pleasant note. This salad is best if tossed together at the last minute.

1½ cups honeydew melon, diced
1½ cups cantaloupe, diced
1 cup fresh peaches, sliced
1 cup seedless grapes
1 cup pitted dates, chopped
¾ cup part-skim mozzarella cheese
½ cup almonds, chopped
⅓ cup honey
⅓ cup frozen limeade concentrate, thawed
1 tablespoon corn oil or safflower oil
2 medium bananas, chopped
Romaine or other lettuce leaves
Fresh strawberries

In a large bowl combine melons, peaches, grapes, dates, cheese and almonds; toss lightly. In a mixer bowl combine honey, limeade concentrate and oil. Beat until whipped. Add with bananas to fruit mixture; toss lightly. In a salad bowl arrange lining of romaine leaves. Spoon salad into the prepared bowl. Garnish with strawberries. Makes 12 servings.

Approx. per serving: 180.0 calories; 5.4 gr. fat; 27.0% calories from fat.

BULGUR-CABBAGE SALAD

Whole wheat kernels that are first steamed, dried and then crushed are called "bulgur." It is a staple grain of the Middle East where it is prized for its delicious nutty flavor. Try this salad stuffed into pita bread.

1 cup water
½ cup bulgur wheat
½ teaspoon salt (optional)
½ cup lite mayonnaise
3 tablespoons cider vinegar
2 tablespoons granulated sugar
½ teaspoon fresh dill or
  ¼ teaspoon dried dillweed
  (optional)
¼ teaspoon Tabasco sauce
  (optional)
¼ teaspoon Dijon mustard
  (optional)
½ cup green onions, thinly sliced
1½ cups cabbage, finely
  shredded
½ cup celery, thinly sliced
½ cup carrot, shredded

In a saucepan combine water, bulgur and salt. Bring to a boil over medium-high heat; stir, cover and reduce heat. Simmer for 15 minutes. In a small bowl combine mayonnaise, vinegar, sugar, dill, Tabasco sauce and mustard; blend well. Stir in green onions. Add to hot cooked bulgur; mix well. Cover. Chill until 1 hour before serving. Add cabbage, celery and carrot; mix well. Cover. Chill until serving time.
Makes 4 to 6 servings.

Approx. per serving: 199.0 calories; 8.4 gr. fat; 37.98% calories from fat; high vitamin A.

MEDITERRANEAN TABBOULEH SALAD

This Mediterranean salad is a favorite summer salad. It's delicious as part of a salad plate for picnics or lunches, and it keeps well in the refrigerator. Bulgur wheat adds a nutty flavor and texture, and fresh mint lends a special touch. If mint isn't in season, simply omit it.

1 cup bulgur wheat
¼ cup olive oil
¼ cup fresh lemon juice
2 cups fresh parsley, chopped
  and lightly packed
1 cup green onions, finely
  chopped
¼ cup fresh mint, chopped
3 tomatoes, diced
1 cucumber, peeled, seeded and
  chopped
1 teaspoon salt (optional)
Freshly ground pepper to taste

In a bowl combine bulgur with enough water to cover. Let stand for 1 hour. Drain well. Add oil and lemon juice; mix lightly. Add parsley, tomatoes, green onions, cucumber and mint; toss to mix. Cover. Chill for 1 hour to overnight. Add salt and pepper; mix lightly. Makes 10 (⅔-cup) servings.

Approx. per serving: 129.0 calories; 5.8 gr. fat; 40.46% calories from fat.

MINESTRONE SALAD

This is perfect summer fare, a one dish meal that is quick to cook and easy to serve. Crusty bread is all you need to accompany this salad.

**12 ounces whole wheat
  elbow pasta
1 tablespoon fresh lemon juice
1 can (16 ounces) Great Northern
  beans, drained and rinsed
1 ½ cups no-oil Italian salad
  dressing
2 cups fresh broccoli florets
1 cup zucchini, cut into rounds
  and sliced into strips
1 cup fresh carrots, cut into rounds
½ cup green onions with tops,
  chopped
½ cup red and/or green bell
  pepper, chopped
Lettuce leaves
Tomato slices**

Cook pasta according to package directions, adding lemon juice to water; drain. In a large bowl mix pasta with beans and salad dressing. Refrigerate overnight. In a saucepan or steamer steam broccoli until tender-crisp. Into a bowl of ice water place broccoli immediately to stop cooking process; drain well. To pasta mixture add broccoli, zucchini, carrots, green onions and bell pepper; mix gently. Let stand for 2 to 3 hours before serving. On salad plates arrange lettuce. Spoon salad onto prepared plates. Garnish with tomato slices. Makes 8 servings.

Approx. per serving: 326.0 calories; 6.0 gr. fat; 16.56% calories from fat; high vitamin A; high fiber.

PASTA BROCCOLI SALAD

Light and refreshing pasta salad has contrasting textures and tastes. Be sure to cook the pasta just until al dente (tender to the bite).

**1 large bunch broccoli
2 cups cooked whole wheat
  fusilli or shell pasta, drained
1 large red bell pepper, seeded
  and sliced
2 stalks celery, chopped
1 medium yellow squash,
  chopped
½ cup scallions, chopped
½ cup cherry tomato halves**

Divide broccoli into florets; peel and slice stems. In a large bowl combine pasta, broccoli, red pepper, celery, squash, scallions and cherry tomatoes. Add dressing; toss until mixed. Chill salad slightly.

Dressing
**⅓ cup white wine vinegar
2 tablespoons olive oil
2 tablespoons fresh lemon juice
2 tablespoons fresh parsley,
  minced
1 tablespoon fresh basil, chopped
  or ½ teaspoon dried basil
1 teaspoon dry mustard
1 clove garlic, pressed**

In a small bowl combine vinegar, olive oil, lemon juice, parsley, basil, dry mustard and garlic; whisk until blended.
Makes 6 to 8 servings.

Approx. per serving: 137.0 calories; 5.0 gr. fat; 32.84% calories from fat.

WILD RICE SALAD

The nutty, distinctive flavor of this grain (which is the seed of a wild grass) is particularly apparent in this scrumptious salad.

½ cup uncooked wild rice
2½ cups water, divided
½ cup long grain white rice
1 slice lemon
1 medium carrot, peeled, trimmed
   and diced
½ green bell pepper, cored,
   seeded and diced
½ red bell pepper, cored, seeded
   and diced
½ cup fresh or frozen green peas
1 stalk celery, washed and
   thinly sliced
3 green onions, washed, trimmed
   and thinly sliced
Chopped parsley

In a bowl place wild rice. Add hot water to cover. Let stand for 1 hour; drain. In a saucepan bring 1½ cups water to a boil; add wild rice. Cover. Cook over medium heat for 20 minutes. Into a colander pour wild rice; rinse under hot running water, shaking occasionally. Drain well. In a saucepan bring 1 cup water to a boil; add long grain rice and lemon slice. Cover. Cook over medium heat for 20 minutes. Into a colander pour the rice; rinse under hot running water, shaking occasionally. Drain well. In a large bowl combine rices. Keep the vegetables separate. In a saucepan cook carrot in boiling water to just cover for 8 to 10 minutes or until just tender. In a colander drain carrot; rinse under cold water. Into a saucepan of boiling water place peppers 1 at a time. Cook each for 1 minute. Drain and rinse with cold water. Add cooked carrot, blanched peppers, peas, celery and green onions to rice mixture. Add dressing; mix well.

Let stand for 1 hour or longer. Into a clear glass bowl spoon the salad. Garnish with chopped parsley. Makes 6 to 8 servings.

Vinaigrette Dressing
¼ cup cider vinegar
1 teaspoon Dijon mustard
2 tablespoons safflower oil
1 teaspoon fresh thyme or
   ½ teaspoon dried thyme

In a small bowl combine vinegar and mustard. Whisk in oil 1 drop at a time. Stir in thyme.

Approx. per serving: 135.0 calories; 5.0 gr. fat; 33.33% calories from fat.

RICE SALAD

With the addition of some cooked seafood or poultry, this could be served as a light entrée.

3 cups cooked brown rice, cooled
3 tablespoons vegetable or
   chicken broth, either
   homemade or canned
2 tablespoons lite mayonnaise
1 teaspoon Dijon mustard
½ teaspoon salt (optional)
¼ teaspoon pepper
⅓ cup scallions, sliced
½ cup green bell pepper, chopped
1 hard-boiled egg, chopped
1 tablespoon capers, drained

In a large bowl combine rice, broth, mayonnaise, mustard, salt and pepper; toss lightly until well mixed. Add scallions, green pepper, egg and capers; toss to mix. Chill until serving time. Makes 8 servings.

Approx. per serving: 135.0 calories; 4.67 gr. fat; 31.33% calories from fat.

ALMOND CHICKEN SALAD

This light elegant entrée is economical and extravagantly good. It begins with chicken breasts simmered until tender and then combined with mayonnaise and tangy yogurt. A light shower of almonds provides the "special" finish.

4 cups cooked skinless, boneless chicken breast, chopped
1 cup celery, chopped
1 cup seedless green grape halves
1 teaspoon salt (optional)
¼ teaspoon pepper
½ cup lite mayonnaise
½ cup low-fat plain yogurt
¼ cup almonds, chopped
Lettuce

In a large bowl combine chicken, celery, grapes, salt and pepper. In a small bowl blend mayonnaise and yogurt. Add to chicken mixture; toss to mix. Chill for several hours. Add almonds just before serving; toss lightly. On salad plates arrange lettuce. Spoon salad onto the prepared plates. Makes 8 to 10 servings.

Approx. per serving: 189.0 calories; 8.7 gr. fat; 41.42% calories from fat.

CHICKEN AND MELON SALAD

1 small honeydew or cantaloupe
6 cups cooked skinless chicken, cubed
2 cups celery, chopped
2 cups seedless green or red grapes
1 cup water chestnuts, sliced (optional)
½ cup low-fat cottage cheese
1 to 2 tablespoons 1% low-fat milk
½ cup low-fat plain yogurt
1 teaspoon curry powder
Salt and freshly ground pepper to taste

Cut melon into halves; discard seed. With a melon baller scoop out pulp. In a large bowl combine melon balls, chicken, celery, grapes and water chestnuts. In a blender container place cottage cheese. Process until smooth, adding enough milk to make of desired consistency. In a small bowl combine blended cottage cheese, yogurt and curry powder; blend well. Add to chicken mixture; mix gently. Season with salt and pepper. Makes 10 cups.

Approx. per cup: 146.0 calories; 2.4 gr. fat; 14.79% calories from fat.

MEXICAN CHICKEN SALAD

Try this South-of-the-Border salad tucked into a fresh corn tortilla.

1 medium head lettuce
1 can (15 ounces) kidney beans, drained
1 cup cooked skinless chicken, chopped
½ cup green bell pepper, chopped
2 scallions, chopped
⅓ cup fresh cilantro (coriander), chopped
3 tablespoons chicken broth, either homemade or canned
2 tablespoons corn oil or safflower oil
2 tablespoons red wine vinegar
1 tablespoon fresh lime juice
1½ teaspoons granulated sugar
1 clove of garlic, minced
¾ teaspoon chili powder
½ teaspoon salt (optional)

Rinse lettuce; drain, pat dry and shred. Into a salad bowl place lettuce, beans, chicken, green pepper and scallions. In a blender container combine cilantro, broth, oil, vinegar, lime juice, sugar, garlic, chili powder and salt. Process until well mixed. Pour over chicken mixture just before serving; toss lightly. Makes 8 servings.

Approx. per serving: 138.0 calories; 4.5 gr. fat; 29.34% calories from fat; high fiber.

TUNA PASTA SALAD

2 cups fettuccine, curly spinach noodles or vegetable non-egg noodles
1 can (7 ounces) water-pack white tuna or albacore, drained
1 can (7 ounces) water chestnuts, diced
4 green onions, diced
1 stalk celery, diced
½ cup low-fat plain yogurt
¼ cup lite mayonnaise
1 tablespoon lite soy sauce
1 clove garlic, finely minced
1 teaspoon fresh parsley or ½ teaspoon dried parsley

Cook and drain fettuccine using package directions. In a large bowl combine fettuccine, tuna, water chestnuts, green onions and celery. In a small bowl combine yogurt, mayonnaise, soy sauce, garlic and parsley; mix well. Add to tuna mixture; toss lightly. Chill in refrigerator. Makes 4 servings.

Approx. per serving: 407.0 calories; 6.4 gr. fat; 14.15% calories from fat.

SALAD NIÇOISE

Tuna, tomatoes, potatoes, green beans, hard-boiled eggs are the usual components for this appetizing salad from the south of France. Serve as an hors d'oeuvre or as a main-course summer salad.

**1 large head romaine lettuce
3 medium new potatoes
  (red preferred)
½ pound fresh green beans
¼ cup red wine vinegar
5 tablespoons vegetable or
  chicken broth, either
  homemade or canned
1½ scallions, sliced
2 tablespoons olive oil
1½ teaspoons Dijon mustard
½ teaspoon salt (optional)
¼ teaspoon pepper
Lettuce leaves
2 cans (7 ounces each)
  water-pack tuna (albacore
  preferred)
3 medium tomatoes, quartered
1 hard-boiled egg, chopped
1 tablespoon capers, drained
12 radishes, washed and sliced
½ cup parsley sprigs**

Rinse and drain lettuce. Refrigerate until crisp. In a saucepan or steamer over medium heat cook potatoes in water to cover until tender; drain and cut into bite-sized pieces. In a bowl place potatoes. In a saucepan or steamer steam green beans until tender-crisp; cut into bite-sized pieces. In a bowl place green beans. In a small bowl combine vinegar, broth, scallions, olive oil, mustard, salt and pepper; mix well. Pour half the dressing over potatoes; pour remaining half over green beans. Marinate for 1 hour or longer. Drain potatoes and green beans, reserving dressing. On a serving platter arrange lettuce leaves to cover. Mound potatoes in center; arrange green beans in circle around potatoes and tuna in circle around beans. Place tomato quarters, egg, capers, radishes and parsley around edge according to your visual taste and the shape of the platter. Drizzle reserved dressing over all. Serve immediately. Makes 10 servings.

Approx. per serving: 187.0 calories; 5.49 gr. fat; 26.42% calories from fat.

ARTICHOKE-TOMATO SALAD

**1 tablespoon red wine vinegar
½ teaspoon Dijon mustard
1 clove garlic, minced
2 tablespoons olive oil
4 green onions, chopped
1 cucumber, coarsely chopped
5 tomatoes, coarsely chopped
1 can (14 ounces) artichoke
  hearts, drained and quartered
1 hard-boiled egg, grated
Salt, freshly ground pepper and
  fresh lemon juice to taste**

In a large salad bowl combine vinegar, mustard and garlic. Whisk in olive oil gradually. Layer green onions, cucumber, tomatoes and artichoke hearts in order listed in prepared bowl. Sprinkle egg over top. Cover. Refrigerate until 15 minutes before serving time. Add salt, pepper and lemon juice; toss lightly. Makes 6 cups.

Approx. per cup: 87.0 calories; 5.7 gr. fat; 58.96% calories from fat.

MARINATED BLACK BEAN SALAD

1 pound dried black beans
3 cups cooked brown rice
1 cup onion, chopped
1 cup green bell pepper, chopped
¼ cup fresh cilantro (coriander) or
  parsley, chopped
3 tablespoons corn oil or
  safflower oil
3 tablespoons red wine vinegar
3 tablespoons vegetable or
  chicken broth, either
  homemade or canned
2 teaspoons fresh thyme or
  1 teaspoon dried thyme
2 cloves garlic, minced
½ teaspoon pepper

Cook beans according to package directions; drain well. In a large bowl place beans, rice, onion and green pepper. In a small bowl place cilantro, oil, vinegar, broth, thyme, garlic and pepper; mix well. Add to bean mixture; toss gently. Marinate in refrigerator for several hours. Makes 12 servings.

Approx. per serving: 153.0 calories; 4.14 gr. fat; 24.35% calories from fat; high fiber.

GARBANZO BEAN SALAD

This delightful concoction makes a good first course arranged on lettuce leaves, or a good accompaniment to simple broiled chicken.

½ pound dried garbanzo beans
½ cup celery, chopped
½ cup green bell pepper, chopped
½ cup green onions, sliced
¼ cup fresh parsley, chopped
1 jar (2 ounces) diced pimento,
  drained
⅔ cup reduced-calorie Italian
  salad dressing
¼ teaspoon pepper, freshly ground
Lettuce leaves

Sort and wash beans. In a large heavy saucepan place beans. Add enough water to cover by 2 inches. Let stand overnight. Drain. Add water to cover. Bring to a boil over medium-high heat; reduce heat. Cover. Simmer for 1 hour or until beans are tender. Drain and cool. In a large bowl combine beans, celery, green pepper, green onions, parsley and pimento. Add salad dressing and pepper; mix well. Cover. Chill for several hours to overnight, stirring occasionally. On salad plates arrange lettuce leaves. Onto lettuce leaves spoon salad using slotted spoon. Makes 8 servings.

Approx. per serving: 137.0 calories; 4.1 gr. fat; 26.9% calories from fat; high fiber.

WHITE BEAN, RED ONION AND TOMATO SALAD

2 cups cooked white beans, tender yet firm
2 tablespoons olive oil
Salt and freshly ground pepper to taste
2 large ripe tomatoes, seeded and diced
¼ cup red onion, finely diced
2 tablespoons fresh oregano or 2 teaspoons dried oregano

In a small bowl place beans. Add olive oil, salt and pepper; mix gently. Add tomatoes, onion and oregano; toss to mix.
Makes 4 servings.

Approx. per serving: 189.0 calories; 7.4 gr. fat; 35.23% calories from fat; high fiber.

BLACK-EYED PEAS VINAIGRETTE

Black-eyed peas (sometimes called cow-peas because of their original use as animal feed) have long been a staple in the South. They add an earthy taste to this appetizing salad. Be sure to add the beans to the vinaigrette while they are hot so they will absorb the flavor.

1 pound dried black-eyed peas
¼ cup vegetable or skimmed chicken broth, either homemade or canned
¼ cup red wine vinegar
2 tablespoons olive oil
2 tablespoons fresh oregano, chopped or 1 tablespoon dried oregano
1½ teaspoons Dijon mustard
2 cloves garlic, minced
1 teaspoon salt (optional)
½ teaspoon pepper
1 cup fresh carrots, grated
1 cup onion, chopped
1 cup fresh parsley, chopped

Cook black-eyed peas according to package directions. In a small bowl combine broth, vinegar, olive oil, oregano, mustard, garlic, salt and pepper; mix well. Let stand while peas cook. Drain peas. In a large bowl combine hot black-eyed peas, carrots, onion and parsley; toss to mix. Add dressing; toss until coated. Cover. Marinate in refrigerator for several hours to overnight. Makes 12 servings.

Approx. per serving: 78.9 calories; 2.47 gr. fat; 28.17% calories from fat; high fiber.

ORIENTAL BEAN SPROUT AND MUSHROOM SALAD

This salad has a delicious, slightly nutty flavor thanks to the sesame seed tossed over the crunchy snow peas and water chestnuts.

1 tablespoon corn oil margarine
2 bunches scallions, sliced
½ pound fresh mushrooms, sliced
¼ pound fresh snow peas
1 pound fresh bean sprouts
4 cups boiling water
2 tablespoons lite soy sauce
2 teaspoons corn oil or safflower oil
2 teaspoons granulated sugar
1 can (7 ounces) sliced water chestnuts, drained
2 tablespoons sesame seed

In a skillet melt margarine over low heat. Add scallions. Sauté for 1 minute. Add mushrooms and snow peas. Sauté just until wilted. Into a colander place bean sprouts. Pour boiling water over sprouts; drain. In a large bowl combine sautéed vegetables and bean sprouts. In a small bowl combine soy sauce, oil and sugar; mix well. Pour over vegetables. Add water chestnuts and sesame seed; toss to mix. Chill until serving time. Makes 6 servings.

Approx. per serving: 106.0 calories; 5.3 gr. fat; 45.0% calories from fat; high fiber.

LEMON-BROCCOLI SALAD

Almost any vegetable could be prepared in this manner—cauliflower, string beans, carrots or mushrooms. Make up a colorful combination for an attractive appetizer, picnic fare or accompaniment to a main course.

2 pounds fresh broccoli
3 tablespoons vegetable or chicken broth, either homemade or canned
3 tablespoons fresh lemon juice
1 ½ tablespoons olive oil
½ teaspoon salt (optional)
¼ teaspoon pepper

Separate broccoli into florets, peel stems and slice crosswise. In a covered saucepan over medium heat steam broccoli in a small amount of water for 5 minutes or until tender-crisp. Drain, reserving liquid for soup. Into a bowl of ice water plunge broccoli immediately to stop cooking process. Drain. In a blender container combine broth, lemon juice, olive oil, salt and pepper. Process until mixed. In a salad bowl place broccoli. Add dressing; toss to coat. Marinate in refrigerator for several hours. Makes 6 servings.

Approx. per serving: 74.0 calories; 3.9 gr. fat; 47.43% calories from fat; high fiber.

COLESLAW DIJON

Our version of a delicatessen favorite with a new twist.

6 cups cabbage, grated
3 cups fresh or frozen corn, cooked and drained
2 carrots, grated
2 stalks celery, sliced
¼ cup vegetable or chicken broth, either homemade or canned
2 tablespoons corn oil or safflower oil
2 tablespoons white wine vinegar
2 teaspoons Dijon mustard
½ teaspoon salt (optional)
½ teaspoon celery seed
2 scallions, sliced

In a large bowl combine cabbage, corn, carrots and celery. In a small bowl combine broth, oil, vinegar, mustard, salt and celery seed; mix well. Stir in scallions. Add to cabbage mixture; toss gently to mix. Chill for several hours to allow flavors to develop. Makes 12 servings.

Approx. per serving: 70.1 calories; 2.67 gr. fat; 34.27% calories from fat; high fiber.

NAPA ORIENTAL SLAW

Napa cabbage is a soft green and off-white leafy vegetable which looks like a pale and compact head of romaine lettuce. The flavor is a delightful combination of mild cabbage, iceberg lettuce and celery. Small heads have the best flavor.

1 medium head Napa (Chinese) cabbage
2 tablespoons salt
2 or 3 carrots, shredded
2 tablespoons corn oil or safflower oil
2 tablespoons water
½ cup green onions, chopped
1 teaspoon fresh gingerroot, minced
¼ cup granulated sugar
¼ cup red wine vinegar
1 teaspoon dried red pepper, crushed

Cut core from cabbage; rinse and drain leaves. Cut leaves into shreds. In a large bowl place shredded cabbage. Sprinkle with salt; add water to cover. Let stand for 1 hour. Drain and rinse cabbage; squeeze dry. On a platter place shredded cabbage; sprinkle with carrots. In a saucepan heat oil and 2 tablespoons water over medium heat. Add green onions and gingerroot. Cook for 2 minutes. In a small bowl mix sugar and vinegar. Add to green onion mixture with red pepper. Pour over cabbage and carrots; toss lightly. Makes 4 to 6 servings.

Approx. per serving: 158.0 calories; 5.0 gr. fat; 28.48% calories from fat; high vitamin A; high fiber.

CARROT AND ORANGE SALAD

4 carrots, grated
2 oranges, sectioned and
cut into bite-sized pieces
2 cups watercress, chopped
3 tablespoons white wine vinegar
3 tablespoons orange juice
1 tablespoon olive oil
1 tablespoon honey
1 ½ teaspoons Dijon mustard
¼ teaspoon salt (optional)

In a bowl place carrots. Add boiling water to cover. Let stand for 5 minutes. Drain, reserving liquid; squeeze carrots dry. Reserved liquid may be used for soup. Cool carrots. In a bowl combine carrots and oranges. Rinse watercress; pat dry. Discard stems; chop watercress. Mix with carrots and oranges. In a small bowl combine vinegar, orange juice, olive oil, honey, mustard and salt; mix well. Pour over carrot mixture; mix well. Marinate for 2 hours or longer. Makes 6 servings.

Approx. per serving: 73.8 calories; 2.41 gr. fat; 29.39% calories from fat; high vitamin A.

RAINBOW SWEET AND SOUR SLAW

¾ cup vinegar
¼ cup corn oil or safflower oil
½ cup granulated sugar
¼ cup onion, finely chopped
⅛ teaspoon salt (optional)
⅛ teaspoon pepper
1 medium head cabbage, shredded

In a small bowl combine vinegar, oil, sugar, onion, salt and pepper; mix well. In a large bowl place cabbage. Add dressing; toss to mix. Makes 6 to 8 servings.

Approx. per serving: 172.0 calories; 9.3 gr. fat; 48.66% calories from fat.

DILLED CARROTS

1 ½ pounds carrots, sliced
¼ cup fresh parsley, chopped
3 tablespoons vegetable or
  chicken broth, either
  homemade or canned
2 tablespoons white wine vinegar
1 tablespoon olive oil
2 teaspoons granulated sugar
2 teaspoons fresh dill, chopped or
  1 teaspoon dried dillweed
½ teaspoon salt (optional)
¼ teaspoon pepper

In a saucepan over medium heat steam carrots until tender-crisp. Drain, reserving liquid for soup. Into a large bowl place carrots. In a small bowl combine parsley, broth, vinegar, olive oil, sugar, dill, salt and pepper; mix well. Pour over warm carrots. Marinate in refrigerator for several hours. Makes 6 servings.

Approx. per serving: 67.1 calories; 2.51 gr. fat; 33.66% calories from fat; high vitamin A; high fiber.

VERY ORANGE SALAD

A simple salad in which the sweetness of the raisins balances the tartness of yogurt and citrus. The carrots provide lots of betacarotene (used to form vitamin A in our bodies) and the orange adds some vitamin C.

2 cups carrots, shredded
1 orange, peeled and chopped
¼ cup orange juice
2 tablespoons low-fat
  plain yogurt
2 tablespoons raisins
Dash of freshly grated nutmeg
Spinach or lettuce leaves

In a medium bowl combine carrots and orange. In a small bowl combine orange juice and yogurt; mix well. Pour over carrot and orange mixture. Add raisins and nutmeg; toss to mix. Chill in refrigerator. On serving plates arrange spinach leaves. Spoon salad onto the prepared plates. Makes 4 (½ to ¾-cup) servings.

Approx. per serving: 64.5 calories; 0.3 gr. fat; 4.18% calories from fat; high vitamin A.

DANISH CUCUMBER SALAD

2 cucumbers
1 tablespoon salt
1 red onion, sliced
¾ cup vinegar
¼ cup granulated sugar
Salt and freshly ground pepper
  to taste
Fresh dill, chopped

Slice unpeeled cucumbers thinly. In a bowl or sieve place cucumber slices. Sprinkle with 1 tablespoon salt. Let stand for 1 hour. Drain and pat cucumber slices dry. Into a bowl place cucumber and red onion slices. In a small saucepan or microwave-safe dish combine vinegar and sugar. Cook over low heat, stirring constantly or heat in microwave until sugar is dissolved. Cool. Pour over cucumbers. Let stand for 30 to 60 minutes. Drain. Into a salad bowl place cucumber slices. Season with salt and pepper. Garnish with dill.
Makes 6 to 8 servings.

Approx. per serving: 52.6 calories; 0.2 gr. fat; 3.42% calories from fat.

RED POTATO SALAD WITH CHIVES

6 medium-large red skin potatoes
½ cup low-fat cottage cheese
½ cup low-fat plain yogurt
¼ cup fresh chives or
  green onions, finely chopped
1 teaspoon salt (optional)
Freshly ground pepper to taste

Scrub potatoes; do not peel. Cut into halves or quarters. In a large saucepan place potatoes with water to cover. Cook over medium heat until tender; drain. Place potatoes in saucepan over medium heat for several seconds, shaking pan constantly until potatoes are dry. Cut into ½-inch cubes. Cool. In a blender container combine cottage cheese and yogurt. Process until creamy. In a large bowl combine potatoes, cottage cheese mixture, chives, salt and pepper; toss to mix. Chill until serving time.
Makes 10 (½-cup) servings.

Approx. per serving: 89.0 calories; 0.5 gr. fat; 5.05% calories from fat.

SPINACH AND GRAPEFRUIT SALAD

An updated version of the standard spinach salad. We've added tart grapefruit and sweet honey and a sprinkling of crunchy sesame seed.

2 large bunches fresh spinach
3 medium red grapefruit
1 tablespoon sesame seed
2 tablespoons vegetable or chicken broth, either homemade or canned
1 tablespoon corn oil or safflower oil
1 tablespoon white wine vinegar
1 tablespoon fresh lemon juice
1 tablespoon honey
¼ teaspoon salt (optional)
¼ teaspoon pepper

W ash spinach; pat dry and discard stems. Peel and section grapefruit; cut into bite-sized pieces. In an ungreased skillet over medium heat toast sesame seed until golden brown, tossing frequently. In a blender container combine broth, oil, vinegar, lemon juice, honey, salt and pepper. Process until mixed. In a salad bowl combine spinach and grapefruit. Add dressing; toss to mix. Sprinkle with sesame seed. Makes 8 servings.

Approx. per serving: 79.6 calories; 2.63 gr. fat; 29.73% calories from fat; high vitamin A; high fiber.

SPINACH-MUSHROOM SALAD

1 pound fresh spinach leaves, washed, dried and torn into bite-sized pieces
½ pound fresh mushrooms, sliced
⅓ cup red wine vinegar
1 tablespoon Worcestershire sauce
2 teaspoons corn oil or safflower oil
1 clove garlic, crushed
¼ teaspoon pepper, freshly ground
1 hard-boiled egg, chopped

I n a large salad bowl combine spinach and mushrooms; set aside. In a small saucepan combine vinegar, Worcestershire sauce, oil, garlic and pepper. Bring to a boil over medium-high heat; remove from heat. Cool. Pour dressing over spinach and mushrooms; toss to mix. Garnish with egg. Serve immediately. Makes 6 servings.

Approx. per serving: 53.7 calories; 2.9 gr. fat; 48.6% calories from fat; high vitamin A.

SPINACH SALAD SUPREME

2 medium red potatoes
1 large or 2 medium bunches fresh
  spinach
1 hard-boiled egg, chopped
2 tablespoons sunflower seed
1 scallion, sliced
2 carrots, grated

In a small saucepan over medium heat steam potatoes in a small amount of water until tender. Cool. Chop potatoes. Wash and dry spinach. In a plastic bag chill spinach in refrigerator until crisp. On a serving platter place spinach. Over spinach arrange potatoes, egg, sunflower seed, scallion and carrots in a circular pattern. Drizzle dressing over salad. Serve immediately. Makes 6 servings.

Dressing
½ cup low-fat plain yogurt
1 tablespoon red wine vinegar
1 tablespoon scallion, finely
  chopped
½ teaspoon fresh tarragon or
  ¼ teaspoon dried tarragon
½ teaspoon salt (optional)
½ teaspoon granulated sugar
½ teaspoon fresh basil or
  ¼ teaspoon dried basil
¼ teaspoon pepper

In a blender container combine yogurt, vinegar, scallion, tarragon, salt, sugar, basil and pepper. Process until blended.

Approx. per serving: 117.0 calories; 2.94 gr. fat; 22.61% calories from fat; high vitamin A; high fiber.

TOMATO RAITA

1 medium cucumber, peeled
1 teaspoon salt (optional)
2 medium tomatoes, cored,
  cut into ½-inch cubes and
  drained
1 tablespoon onion, finely chopped
1 cup low-fat plain yogurt
¼ cup fresh parsley, chopped
2 tablespoons fresh cilantro
  (coriander), chopped
1 teaspoon cumin

Cut cucumber in half lengthwise; remove seed. Cut into thin slices. Into a bowl place cucumber. Sprinkle with salt. Let stand for 40 minutes. Drain, squeezing cucumber slightly to remove excess moisture. Add tomatoes and onion. In a bowl combine yogurt, parsley, cilantro and cumin; mix well. Pour over vegetables; mix well. Cover. Chill until serving time.
Makes 4 (¾-cup) servings.

Approx. per serving: 61.0 calories; 1.1 gr. fat; 16.22% calories from fat.

JULIENNE VEGETABLES WITH LEMON VINAIGRETTE

White or yellow turnips or tender parsnips cut into julienne strips are delicious additions to this salad.

**1 cup carrots, cut into
  julienne strips
1 cup zucchini, cut into
  julienne strips
1 cup green beans, cut into
  1½-inch pieces
1 cup celery, cut into
  julienne strips
Salt and freshly ground pepper
  to taste**

In a medium bowl combine carrots, zucchini, green beans and celery; toss lightly to mix. Add Lemon Vinaigrette; toss to mix. Add salt and pepper. Cover. Refrigerate until serving time.
Makes 6 (⅔-cup) servings.

Lemon Vinaigrette
**¼ cup fresh lemon juice
2 tablespoons fresh parsley,
  chopped or 1 tablespoon dried
  parsley
2 tablespoons green onion tops or
  fresh chives, chopped
1 tablespoon olive oil
1 clove garlic, minced**

In a small bowl combine lemon juice, parsley, green onion tops, olive oil and garlic; mix well.

Approx. per serving: 44.5 calories; 2.4 gr. fat; 48.53% calories from fat; high vitamin A.

VEGETABLE SALAD

**1 medium head broccoli
1 medium cucumber, peeled,
  grated and drained
2 carrots, grated**

Break broccoli into florets. Peel and thinly slice stems. In a saucepan place broccoli florets and stems. Cover with boiling water. Let stand for 5 minutes. Drain, reserving liquid for soup. In a salad bowl combine broccoli, cucumber and carrots. Add dressing; toss gently. Serve at room temperature or chilled.
Makes 6 servings.

Dressing
**¾ cup low-fat plain yogurt
¼ cup scallions, chopped
¼ cup green bell pepper, chopped
1 tablespoon fresh lemon juice
1 teaspoon fresh dill or
  ½ teaspoon dried dillweed
¼ teaspoon salt (optional)**

In a small bowl combine yogurt, scallions, green pepper, lemon juice, dill and salt; mix well.

Approx. per serving: 46.5 calories; 0.75 gr. fat; 14.51% calories from fat; high vitamin A; high fiber.

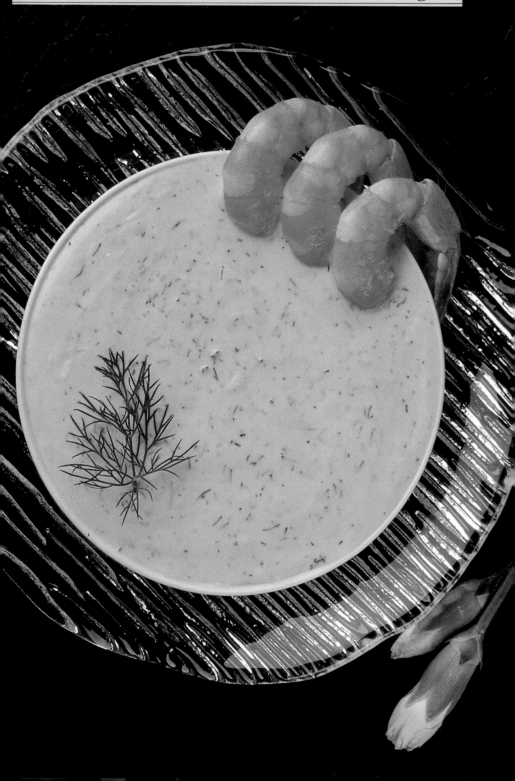

Sauces, salad dressings and spices enhance the food they accompany with flavor, color and texture. Many times they also add unwanted calories, fat and salt. You can duplicate the same wonderful sauces and salad dressings quickly and with fewer calories by using the recipes on the following pages.

Puréed vegetables make a rich, delicious sauce for poultry, pasta, meat or fish. Puréed fruits and berries combined with a small amount of liqueur make terrific low-fat toppings for ice milk, sorbet, sherbet, soufflés or cakes. Use your microwave oven to cook sauces quickly and preserve their nutrients. Try the *Mock Sour Cream* the next time you bake a potato, and see how delicious sauces that are good for you can be. (Real sour cream has 485 calories a cup!)

Salad dressings make wonderful marinades. A quick way of marinating is to place the food in a dish with the marinade and place in the microwave oven set on the lowest power for 1 to 2 minutes before cooking. Variations on your basic vinaigrette dressing can be made by using flavored herb vinegars or fresh herbs, such as basil, tarragon, parsley or chives, and freshly minced garlic can add some zest.

Recipe for this photograph on page 72.

ALL-PURPOSE
ONION SAUCE

2 tablespoons corn oil margarine
2 tablespoons onion, finely
chopped
2 tablespoons all-purpose flour
1 ½ cups vegetable broth, either
homemade or canned
2 teaspoons lite soy sauce
½ teaspoon salt (optional)
Freshly ground pepper to taste

In a saucepan over medium heat melt margarine. Add onion. Cook until light brown. Stir in flour; remove from heat. Stir in broth, soy sauce, salt and pepper. Cook until thickened, stirring constantly. Makes 1½ cups (2 tablespoons per serving).

Approx. per serving: 44.5 calories; 2.2 gr. fat; 44.5% calories from fat.

CHILI
SAUCE

Use on Mexican foods, such as chilies rellenos, burritos and tacos, and to add interest to plain meat or chicken.

1 cup tomato sauce
2 tablespoons red wine vinegar
2 tablespoons mild green chilies,
diced
1½ tablespoons onion,
finely chopped
½ teaspoon cumin, ground

In a small saucepan combine tomato sauce, vinegar, chilies, onion and cumin; mix well. Simmer for 15 minutes. Serve hot. Makes 1⅓ cups.

Approx. per serving: 4.0 calories; 0.02 gr. fat; 4.5% calories from fat.

BEST EVER
BARBECUE SAUCE

This spicy barbecue sauce is so good you'll want to place a bowl on the table so everyone can have extra. To make the sauce real "mean" add a fresh jalapeño pepper, seeded and minced.

3 cups catsup
¾ cup packed light brown sugar
5 teaspoons liquid smoke
1 tablespoon dry mustard

In a small saucepan combine catsup, brown sugar, liquid smoke and dry mustard. Simmer for 10 minutes. Brush on grilled or broiled meats during last 10 to 15 minutes of cooking time. Makes 3 to 4 cups.

Approx. per serving: 28.0 calories; 0.0 gr. fat; 0.0% calories from fat.

CREAMY DILL SAUCE

Although dill has a particularly wonderful affinity for salmon this sauce would be good with any poached or baked fish. Try it as a dip for crudités or as a refreshing salad dressing.

1 cup low-fat plain yogurt
2 tablespoons fresh parsley, finely chopped
2 teaspoons fresh dill, finely chopped
2 teaspoons Dijon mustard
½ teaspoon celery seed
Salt and pepper to taste

In a small bowl combine yogurt, parsley, dill, mustard, celery seed, salt and pepper; mix well. Cover. Chill for 3 hours to 5 days. Stir before serving.
Makes 1 cup
(2 tablespoons per serving).

Approx. per serving: 19.4 calories; 0.52 gr. fat; 24.12% calories from fat.

Photograph for this recipe on page 69.

MARINARA SAUCE

Marinara is a delicious meatless tomato sauce, good with any type of pasta.

1 tablespoon olive oil
½ cup onion, chopped
2 cloves garlic, minced
1 can (14½ ounces) Italian-style tomatoes
1 can (15 ounces) tomato sauce
1 can (6 ounces) tomato paste
½ cup red wine
1 tablespoon fresh basil or
1½ teaspoons dried basil
1½ teaspoons granulated sugar
1 bay leaf
½ teaspoon fresh oregano or
¼ teaspoon dried oregano
¼ teaspoon salt (optional)
¼ teaspoon pepper

In a large saucepan heat olive oil over low heat. Add onion and garlic. Sauté until transparent. In a blender container purée tomatoes with juice. Add to onion mixture. Add tomato sauce, tomato paste, wine, basil, sugar, bay leaf, oregano, salt and pepper; mix well. Simmer, uncovered, for 1 hour. Discard bay leaf. Serve hot over pasta.
Makes 5½ cups (½ cup per serving).

Approx. per serving: 55.0 calories; 1.5 gr. fat; 24.54% calories from fat.

MINT
SAUCE

1 cup low-fat plain yogurt
3 tablespoons fresh lemon juice
2 tablespoons fresh mint, finely
  chopped or 1 tablespoon
  dried mint
1 teaspoon fresh basil or
  ½ teaspoon dried basil
1 clove garlic, minced
½ teaspoon salt (optional)
¼ teaspoon granulated sugar

In the top of a double boiler combine yogurt, lemon juice, mint, basil, garlic, salt and sugar; mix well. In the bottom of the double boiler place a small amount of water. Heat over low heat until hot. Over the hot water place the top of the double boiler. Heat to serving temperature.
Makes 1¼ cups.

Approx. per tablespoon: 7.85 calories; 0.17 gr. fat; 19.49% calories from fat.

TARRAGON AND
MUSHROOM SAUCE

Similar in taste to a Bearnaise sauce but with much less butter, this is delicious served warm with meats of all kinds or with vegetarian main dishes such as lentil burgers.

1 tablespoon corn oil margarine
1 cup fresh mushrooms, chopped
2 tablespoons shallots, chopped
4 teaspoons all-purpose flour
1 teaspoon fresh tarragon or
  ½ teaspoon dried tarragon
2 cups beef broth, either
  homemade or canned

In a small saucepan melt margarine over medium heat. Add mushrooms and shallots. Sauté until vegetables are tender and liquid is almost evaporated. Sprinkle flour and tarragon over vegetables. Cook for 2 minutes, stirring constantly. In a small saucepan over medium heat bring broth to a boil. Add to mushroom mixture gradually, stirring constantly with a wire whisk. Cook until mixture comes to a boil and thickens slightly, stirring constantly. Simmer for 10 to 20 minutes or until sauce is reduced to 1 cup. Serve hot. Makes 1 cup.

Approx. per serving: 24.5 calories; 1.6 gr. fat; 58.77% calories from fat.

THREE-PEPPER SAUCE FOR PASTA

We like to serve this sauce over linguini, spaghetti or fettuccine. Although it is delicious with the traditional sprinkle of Parmesan cheese, try topping with a dollop of Mock Sour Cream and a grinding of black pepper.

2 tablespoons olive oil
2 small green bell peppers,
 cut into julienne strips
1 small yellow bell pepper,
 cut into julienne strips
1 small red bell pepper,
 cut into julienne strips
1 onion, cut into thin strips
1 clove garlic, minced
2 medium tomatoes, cored,
 seeded and diced
6 tablespoons fresh basil, minced
¼ teaspoon salt (optional)
⅛ teaspoon pepper, freshly ground
1 strip orange rind

In a large skillet heat olive oil over medium heat. Add bell peppers, onion and garlic. Sauté for 5 minutes or until tender. Add tomatoes, basil, salt, pepper and orange rind; mix well. Cook, uncovered, until heated through. Makes 8 servings.

Approx. per serving: 53.0 calories; 3.7 gr. fat; 62.83% calories from fat.

HONEY MUSTARD

½ cup Dijon mustard
⅓ cup honey

In a small bowl combine mustard and honey; blend well. Let stand for several hours to blend flavors. Makes ⅔ cup.

Approx. per serving: 38.0 calories; 0.47 gr. fat; 11.13% calories from fat.

MUSTARD AVEC FINES HERBES

3 tablespoons dry mustard
2 tablespoons all-purpose flour
2 tablespoons fresh chives,
 snipped or 1 tablespoon
 dried chives
2 tablespoons fresh chervil or
 1 tablespoon dried chervil
2 tablespoons fresh tarragon or
 1 tablespoon dried tarragon
2 tablespoons fresh parsley,
 minced or 1 tablespoon dried
 parsley flakes
2 teaspoons granulated sugar
½ teaspoon turmeric
½ teaspoon salt (optional)
½ cup water
½ cup dry white wine

In a medium saucepan combine dry mustard, flour, chives, chervil, tarragon, parsley, sugar, turmeric and salt; mix well. Stir in water and wine gradually. Bring to a boil over high heat, stirring constantly. Cook for 1 minute, stirring constantly. Into a jar pour the mustard. Cover tightly. Refrigerate for several hours to allow the flavors to blend. Mix well before serving. Makes 1 cup
(2 tablespoons per serving).

Approx. per serving: 76.5 calories; 0.81 gr. fat; 9.5% calories from fat.

YOGURT HOLLANDAISE

Sauce can be prepared in advance, refrigerated for up to 1 week, then reheated over hot water.

¾ cup egg substitute *
1 cup low-fat plain yogurt
2 teaspoons fresh lemon juice
1 tablespoon fresh dill or
**   parsley, chopped (optional)**
½ teaspoon Dijon mustard
½ teaspoon salt (optional)
Pinch of freshly ground pepper

In the top of a non-aluminum double boiler combine Egg Beaters, yogurt and lemon juice; mix well. In the bottom of the double boiler place a small amount of water. Heat water to the simmering point. Over the simmering water place the top of the double boiler. Cook for about 15 minutes or until thickened, stirring frequently. (Mixture will become thinner after cooking for 10 minutes and will thicken again during remaining cooking time.) Remove from heat. Stir in dill, mustard, salt and pepper.
Make 1¼ cups.
(2 tablespoons per serving).

* Nutritional analysis based on using *Fleischmann's Egg Beaters* egg substitute. Fat and calorie content may vary between brands.

Approx. per serving: 28 calories; 0.9 gr. fat; 28.9% calories from fat.

QUICK AND EASY FRESH APPLESAUCE

A delicious applesauce that tastes just like a fresh apple. It's easy to prepare in either the blender or the food processor.

4 apples, peeled and chopped
½ cup honey
2 tablespoons fresh lemon juice
Cinnamon to taste

In a blender container combine apples, honey, lemon juice and cinnamon. Process until smooth. Into a serving dish pour applesauce. Makes 8 servings.

Approx. per servings: 102.0 calories; 0.2 gr. fat; 1.76% calories from fat.

FRESH PEAR SAUCE

4 very ripe Anjou pears, peeled,
**   cored and cut into 1-inch chunks**
1 vanilla bean, split
1 tablespoon water

In a heavy medium saucepan combine pears, vanilla bean and water; cover. Cook over medium heat for 7 to 10 minutes or until pears yield juice. Uncover. Cook until liquid is reduced to 3 tablespoons, stirring frequently. Into pears scrape seed from vanilla bean; discard pod. Into a food processor place the pears and liquid. Process until puréed. Serve warm or chilled with soufflés or over berries or puddings.
Makes 1 cup.

Approx. per tablespoon: 25.0 calories; 0.16 gr. fat; 5.76% calories from fat.

APPLE AND LEMON SAUCE FOR BROILED CHICKEN

This sauce turns ordinary broiled chicken into a special event.

2 lemons
3 large Golden Delicious or Granny Smith apples, peeled, quartered and cored
3 tablespoons chicken broth, either homemade or canned
Salt and pepper to taste
Cinnamon to taste (optional)

With a vegetable peeler peel zest from lemons in thin strips; remove only yellow rind. Chop zest finely. Into a measuring cup squeeze lemon juice. Reserve ¼ cup juice. In a heavy saucepan place apples and lemon juice; cover. Cook over low heat for 20 minutes. In a small saucepan combine lemon zest and water to cover. Bring to a boil over medium-high heat. Cook for 7 to 8 minutes; drain. In blender container or food processor combine the apples and chicken broth. Process until puréed. In a small bowl combine apple purée, lemon zest, salt, pepper and cinnamon; mix well. Serve hot. Makes 4 servings.

Approx. per serving: 60.0 calories; 0.4 gr. fat; 6.0% calories from fat.

GINGER SAUCE

1 can (16 ounces) juice-pack apricots, pitted
½ cup light corn syrup
¼ cup cider vinegar
¼ cup green onions, sliced
¼ to ½ teaspoon ginger, ground
⅛ teaspoon allspice, ground
⅛ teaspoon cayenne pepper

In a blender container place apricots and juice. Add corn syrup, vinegar, green onions, ginger, allspice and cayenne pepper. Process until smooth. Into a small saucepan pour apricot mixture. Bring to a boil; reduce heat. Simmer for 45 minutes.
Makes 2¾ cups
(¼ cup per serving).

Approx. per serving: 46.0 calories; 0.02 gr. fat; 0.39% calories from fat.

APRICOT DIPPING SAUCE

This makes a great dipping sauce for Oriental appetizers.

1 cup apricot preserves
1½ tablespoons fresh gingerroot, grated
1 tablespoon cider vinegar
1 teaspoon Dijon mustard

In a small saucepan over low heat combine apricot preserves, gingerroot, vinegar and mustard. Heat until preserves melt and ingredients are blended, stirring constantly. Makes 1 cup.

Approx. per tablespoon: 54.0 calories; 0.04 gr. fat; 0.7% calories from fat.

CRANBERRY CATSUP

This spicy condiment is wonderful with turkey, chicken or duck.

1 tablespoon corn oil or safflower oil
1 ½ cups onions, coarsely chopped
3 strips (½ inch wide) orange zest
1 strip (½ inch wide) lemon zest
2 ¼ cups water
1 package (12 ounces) fresh cranberries
½ cup cider vinegar
1 cup packed light brown sugar
¾ teaspoon cinnamon
¾ teaspoon allspice
½ teaspoon salt (optional)
½ teaspoon ginger
½ teaspoon paprika
¼ teaspoon mace
1 small bay leaf
⅛ teaspoon cayenne pepper
Pinch of cloves, ground

In a large non-aluminum saucepan heat oil over low heat. Add onion and orange and lemon zests; cover. Cook for 10 minutes or until soft but not brown. Add water, cranberries and vinegar. Cook over medium heat for 10 minutes or until cranberries pop. Strain, reserving both liquid and cranberries. In a food processor or blender container process cranberries for 30 seconds or until puréed. Into a saucepan place purée and stir in reserved liquid. Add brown sugar, cinnamon, allspice, salt, ginger, paprika, mace, bay leaf, cayenne pepper and cloves. Bring to a boil over medium heat; reduce heat. Simmer for about 40 minutes or until thickened. Into a jar ladle the catsup; cover tightly. In the refrigerator store for up to 2 weeks. Makes 6 cups (2 tablespoons per serving).

Approx. per serving: 25.79 calories; 0.32 gr. fat; 11.2% calories from fat.

GINGER SAUCE FOR FRUIT

2 cups low-fat plain yogurt
1 tablespoon light brown sugar
1 teaspoon crystallized ginger, chopped

In a small bowl combine yogurt, brown sugar and ginger; mix well. Serve with fresh berries or fruit. Makes 1 cup.

Approx. per serving: 48.0 calories; 0.9 gr. fat; 16.87% calories from fat.

STRAWBERRY SAUCE FOR FRUIT

Berries are wonderful to eat as they are, but when puréed with a little Grand Marnier and sugar they make a superb topping for other fruits, sorbets or soufflés. Raspberries can be substituted for the strawberries.

1 pint fresh strawberries, washed, hulled and sliced
3 tablespoons granulated sugar
1 teaspoon Grand Marnier

In a bowl place strawberries. Sprinkle with sugar and Grand Marnier. Let stand at room temperature for 1 hour. In a blender or food processor process strawberries until puréed. Into a bowl or freezer container place strawberry sauce. Store in refrigerator for 2 to 3 weeks or in freezer for 3 to 4 months. Makes 8 servings.

Approx. per serving: 34.0 calories; 0.13 gr. fat; 3.44% calories from fat.

SPICE BLEND NUMBER 1

Try using this spice blend in place of salt.

1½ teaspoons pepper
1 teaspoon dry mustard
1 teaspoon onion powder
1 teaspoon paprika
1 teaspoon garlic powder
1 teaspoon dried thyme (optional)
¼ teaspoon dried basil

In a bowl combine pepper, dry mustard, onion powder, paprika, garlic powder, thyme and basil; mix well. Into a small tightly covered jar place mixture. Store in a cool dry place.
Makes 6¾ teaspoons.

Approx. per teaspoon: 5.0 calories; 0.0 gr. fat; 0.0% calories from fat.

SPICE BLEND NUMBER 2

This spice blend can be used in cooking as well as at the table.

4 teaspoons onion powder
4 teaspoons paprika
4 teaspoons parsley flakes
2 teaspoons garlic powder
1 teaspoon dried basil

In a bowl combine onion powder, paprika, parsley flakes, garlic powder and basil; mix well. Into a small tightly covered jar place mixture. Store in a cool dry place.
Makes 5 tablespoons.

Approx. per tablespoon: 14.6 calories; 0.24 gr. fat; 14.79% calories from fat.

ZESTY SEASONING MIX

½ cup mustard seed
½ cup white peppercorns
3 tablespoons red pepper, crushed
8 bay leaves, broken into small pieces

In a small jar combine mustard seed, peppercorns, red pepper and bay leaves. Cover tightly; shake until well mixed. Use in preparing pickles, relishes, sauces, stews or soups. For a Hot Mary drink combine 1 cup tomato juice and ¾ teaspoon mix in a saucepan; cover. Simmer for 5 minutes. Into a mug strain the tomato juice. Add vodka to taste and garnish with a lemon wedge.
Makes 20 tablespoons.

Approx. per tablespoon: 35.0 calories; 1.5 gr. fat; 38.57% calories from fat.

CHINESE FIVE-SPICE POWDER

Kept in a tightly closed container this five-spice powder should keep for 6 months.

1 teaspoon cinnamon, ground
1 teaspoon aniseed, crushed
¼ teaspoon fennel seed, crushed
¼ teaspoon pepper, freshly ground
⅛ teaspoon cloves, ground

In a blender combine cinnamon, aniseed, fennel seed, pepper and cloves. Process until powdered. In a tightly covered jar store seasoning in a cool dry place. Season stir-fried vegetables with ¼ to ½ teaspoon seasoning.
Makes 2½ teaspoons.

Approx. per teaspoon: 3.4 calories; 0.11 gr. fat; 29.1% calories from fat.

MAKE-YOUR-OWN CURRY POWDER

¼ cup coriander seed
¼ cup turmeric, ground
4 inches stick cinnamon, broken
1 tablespoon cumin seed
1 teaspoon cardamom seed
1 teaspoon black peppercorns
1 teaspoon ginger, ground
5 whole cloves
2 bay leaves

Preheat oven to 200 degrees. In a shallow baking pan combine coriander, turmeric, cinnamon, cumin seed, cardamom, peppercorns, ginger, cloves and bay leaves. Bake for 25 minutes, stirring occasionally. Into a blender container place the spice mixture. Process until finely ground. Into small jars divide mixture into ¼ cup portions; seal tightly.
Makes 3 (¼-cup) portions.

Approx. per portion: 16.6 calories; 0.51 gr. fat; 27.0% calories from fat.

FRUIT VINEGAR

Can be used in place of any other vinegar for a truly unique salad dressing. Decorative bottles of this vinegar make beautiful, attractive and delicious gifts.

1½ cups white wine vinegar
1 tablespoon honey
½ cup red seedless grapes
1 thin slice fresh orange
Zest of 1 small orange
Zest of 1 small lemon

In a small saucepan combine vinegar and honey. Heat over low heat until warm. Into a decorative 1-pint bottle drop grapes, orange slice, orange zest and lemon zest. Into fruit-filled bottle pour vinegar mixture. Seal. Let stand for several days.
Makes 1 pint.

Approx. per serving: 3.0 calories; 0.0 gr. fat; 0.0% calories from fat.

GREEN
SALSA

A delicious and colorful variation of the better known red salsa. It is excellent as a dip for tortilla chips, or as a sauce for enchiladas, tacos or any other Mexican dish.

1 can (13 ounces) Mexican green tomatoes (tomatillos), drained and chopped
⅓ cup onion, finely chopped
¼ cup fresh cilantro (coriander), chopped
1 tablespoons corn oil or safflower oil
1½ teaspoons mild green chilies, diced
1 clove garlic, minced
¼ teaspoon salt (optional)
⅛ teaspoon pepper
⅛ teapoon granulated sugar
Tortilla chips

In a blender container or food processor place tomatoes, onion, cilantro, oil, chilies, garlic, salt, pepper and sugar. Process briefly; do not purée. Mixture should have texture. Serve at room temperature or chilled. Serve with tortilla chips. Makes 2 cups (⅓ cup per serving).

Approx. per serving: 36.0 calories; 2.4 gr. fat; 60.0% calories from fat.

RED
SALSA

4 medium firm ripe tomatoes, peeled, seeded and chopped
½ white onion, finely diced
½ cup fresh cilantro (coriander), finely chopped
2 or 3 hot jalapeño or serrano chilies, stemmed, seeded and finely minced
½ teaspoon salt (optional)

In a bowl combine tomatoes, onion, cilantro, chilies and salt; mix well. Salsa should be prepared as close to serving time as possible. Makes 1½ cups (¼ cup per serving).

Approx. per serving: 15.0 calories; 0.14 gr. fat; 8.0% calories from fat.

GRATED CUCUMBER
RELISH

3 medium cucumbers, peeled, seeded and grated
1 tablespoon fresh lemon juice
¼ teaspoon salt (optional)
Freshly ground pepper to taste

In a bowl combine cucumbers, lemon juice, salt and pepper; mix well. Chill in refrigerator until serving time.
Makes 1½ cups
(2 tablespoons per serving).

Approx. per serving: 7.5 calories; 0.025 gr. fat; 3.0% calories from fat.

PEPPER AND CUCUMBER RELISH

This would be a delightful side dish to serve with cold turkey or chicken.

8 cups cucumbers, finely minced
4 cups onions, finely minced
2 green bell peppers,
finely minced
2 red bell peppers,
finely minced
¼ cup salt
2 cups cider vinegar, divided
2½ cups water, divided
3 cups granulated sugar
2 tablespoons white
mustard seed
1½ teaspoons peppercorns
1 teaspoon whole allspice

In a large bowl combine cucumbers, onions and bell peppers. Sprinkle with salt; mix well. Let stand at room temperature overnight. Drain well. In a large saucepan combine 1 cup vinegar and 2 cups water. Add vegetables. Bring to a boil over medium-high heat; reduce heat. Cook for 15 minutes. Drain. Add sugar, mustard seed, peppercorns, allspice, the remaining 1 cup vinegar and ½ cup water. Bring to a boil, stirring constantly. Cook for 15 minutes. Into hot sterilized jars ladle relish, leaving ½-inch headspace. With 2-piece lids seal jars. In a boiling water bath process jars for 10 minutes. Makes 8 pints (¼ cup per serving).

Approx. per serving: 42.0 calories; 0.04 gr. fat; 0.08% calories from fat.

ZUCCHINI-APPLE CHUTNEY

This chunky, low-sodium chutney is sweet, tart and full of flavor. It complements roast meats or poultry, hot or cold.

6 cups zucchini, unpeeled, grated
2 cups tart apples, unpeeled,
grated
¾ pound raisins, ground
1⅓ cups vinegar
1 cup honey
2 green bell peppers,
coarsely ground
1 onion, finely ground
⅓ cup frozen orange juice
concentrate
Juice and grated rind of 1 lemon
1 tablespoon celery seed

In a stockpot combine zucchini, apples, raisins, vinegar, honey, green peppers, onion, orange juice concentrate, lemon juice and rind and celery seed. Simmer until of desired consistency. Into hot sterilized jars ladle chutney, leaving ½-inch headspace. With 2-piece lids seal jars. In a boiling water bath process jars for 10 minutes. Cool. Let stand for 1 to 2 weeks before serving to allow flavors to mellow. Makes 5 cups.

Approx. per serving: 31.7 calories; 0.08 gr. fat; 2.27% calories from fat.

BLUE CHEESE DRESSING

Using yogurt instead of traditional mayonnaise in this dressing makes a lighter but equally good-tasting dressing that is much lower in both fat and calories. Use with green and spinach salads.

⅓ cup blue cheese, crumbled, divided
1 cup low-fat plain yogurt
1 clove garlic, minced
Pinch of dry mustard
Freshly ground pepper to taste

In a small bowl cream half the blue cheese with a fork. Add yogurt, garlic, mustard and pepper; mix well. Stir in remaining blue cheese. Cover. Store in refrigerator. Makes 1⅓ cups.

Approx. per serving: 16.4 calories; 0.9 gr. fat; 49.39% calories from fat.

DILLED CUCUMBER DRESSING

1 cucumber, unpeeled, shredded
½ cup low-fat cottage cheese
½ cup low-fat plain yogurt or skim-milk buttermilk
1 bunch fresh dill or
1 tablespoon dried dillweed
1 clove garlic, minced
1 teaspoon fresh lemon juice
Salt and pepper to taste

In a colander drain cucumber until almost dry. In a blender container combine cucumber, cottage cheese, yogurt, dill, garlic, lemon juice, salt and pepper. Process until blended and smooth. Makes 1 cup.

Approx. per serving: 12.0 calories; 0.2 gr. fat; 15.0% calories from fat.

HERBED BUTTERMILK DRESSING

1 cup low-fat buttermilk
½ cup low-fat plain yogurt
½ cup lite mayonnaise
2 tablespoons fresh dill or
    1 tablespoon dried dillweed
1 tablespoon green onion, minced
1 tablespoon fresh parsley, finely
    minced or ½ tablespoon
    dried parsley
½ teaspoon celery seed

In a mixer bowl or a covered jar combine buttermilk, yogurt, mayonnaise, dill, green onion, parsley and celery seed. Beat or shake until blended. Chill thoroughly before serving. Makes 2¼ cups.

Approx. per serving: 13.7 calories; 1.0 gr. fat; 65.69% calories from fat.

HERBED MAYONNAISE

Our light, low-calorie, low-fat mayonnaise may be flavored to suit the occasion with additional herbs or garlic.

1 cup low-fat plain yogurt
½ cup low-fat cottage cheese
¼ cup fresh parsley, chopped
2 tablespoons green onion,
    chopped
1 tablespoon fresh lemon juice
1 tablespoon Dijon mustard
1 teaspoon fresh basil or
    ½ teaspoon dried basil
¼ teaspoon salt (optional)

In a blender container combine yogurt, cottage cheese, parsley, green onions, lemon juice, mustard, basil and salt. Process until smooth; scrape sides occasionally. Makes 2 cups
(2 tablespoons per serving).

Approx. per serving: 17.2 calories; 0.42 gr. fat; 21.97% calories from fat.

PARSLEY DRESSING

This thick, creamy dressing is one of our favorites. It's excellent with spinach and green salads and can also be served as dip for vegetables.

½ cup fresh parsley, chopped
1 cup low-fat cottage cheese
1 egg*
1 teaspoon Dijon mustard
1 teaspoon fresh lemon juice
Salt and freshly ground pepper
   to taste

In a food processor chop parsley. Add cottage cheese, egg, mustard, lemon juice, and salt and pepper. Process until well mixed. Into a covered refrigerator container pour dressing. Refrigerate until serving time.
Makes 1 cup
(2 tablespoons per serving).

* To reduce fat and cholesterol, use an egg substitute with less than 2 grams fat per serving. Fat and calorie content may vary between brands.

Approx. per serving: 31.0 calories; 1.0 gr. fat; 29.0% calories from fat.

MOCK SOUR CREAM

Our luscious, low-calorie sour cream is just the right topping for baked potatoes.

1 cup low-fat cottage cheese
¼ cup skim-milk buttermilk
½ teaspoon (or more) fresh
   lemon juice

In a blender container combine cottage cheese and buttermilk. Process until smooth. Stir in lemon juice to taste. Makes 1 cup.

Approx. per serving: 9.5 calories; 0.2 gr. fat; 18.94% calories from fat.

STAY-TRIM
DRESSING

This dressing derives its spicy flavor from horseradish and garlic. Prepare the dressing a few hours or a few days before serving to allow the flavors to blend and mellow. It may be stored, tightly covered, for up to 1 week in the refrigerator.

1 teaspoon cornstarch
½ teaspoon dry mustard
1 cup water
¼ cup catsup
2 tablespoons vinegar
½ teaspoon Worcestershire
  sauce
½ teaspoon horseradish
½ teaspoon paprika
1 small clove garlic, crushed

In a small saucepan mix cornstarch and dry mustard. Stir in water gradually. Cook over medium heat until thickened, stirring constantly. Cool. Add catsup, vinegar, Worcestershire sauce, horseradish, paprika and garlic; mix well. Into a small covered jar pour dressing. Store in refrigerator. Shake well before using. Makes 21 tablespoons.

Approx. per tablespoon: 4.0 calories; 0.0 gr. fat; 0.0% calories from fat.

TOMATO
FRENCH DRESSING

½ cup tomato juice
1 teaspoon cornstarch
1 tablespoon red wine vinegar
1 tablespoon olive oil
1 teaspoon fresh tarragon,
  thyme or basil or ½ teaspoon
  dried tarragon, thyme or basil.
½ teaspoon Dijon mustard
1 small clove garlic, minced
Salt and freshly ground pepper
  to taste

In a small saucepan whisk together tomato juice and cornstarch until blended. Cook over medium heat until mixture comes to a boil and thickens, stirring constantly. Boil for 1 minute, stirring constantly. Remove from heat. Whisk in vinegar, olive oil, tarragon, mustard, garlic and salt and pepper. Into a jar pour dressing. Cover tightly. Store in refrigerator. Shake before using. Makes ⅔ cup.

Approx. per tablespoon: 15.0 calories; 1.4 gr. fat; 84.0% calories from fat.

YOGURT-DILL SALAD DRESSING

½ cup low-fat plain yogurt
½ cup 1% low-fat milk
1 tablespoon fresh lemon juice
1 tablespoon fresh dill or
   ½ tablespoon dried dillweed
2 teaspoons onion, grated
½ clove garlic, finely minced
¼ teaspoon fresh oregano or
   ⅛ teaspoon dried oregano
⅛ teaspoon freshly ground pepper

In a blender container combine yogurt, milk, lemon juice, dill, onion, garlic, oregano and pepper. Process until smooth. Refrigerate for 1 hour. Serve over salad greens. Makes 1 cup.

Approx. per tablespoon: 7.4 calories; 0.12 gr. fat; 14.59% calories from fat.

YOGURT AND HONEY POPPY SEED DRESSING

This tart-sweet dressing is fantastic on fruit salads and particularly delectable on spinach salad with rings of purple onion.

1 cup low-fat plain yogurt
⅓ cup honey
4 teaspoons fresh lemon juice
1 teaspoon poppy seed

In a bowl combine yogurt, honey, lemon juice and poppy seed; mix well. Serve over fresh fruit. Makes 1⅓ cups.

Approx. per tablespoon: 22.6 calories; 0.22 gr. fat; 8.76% calories from fat.

Pasta · Rice · Beans

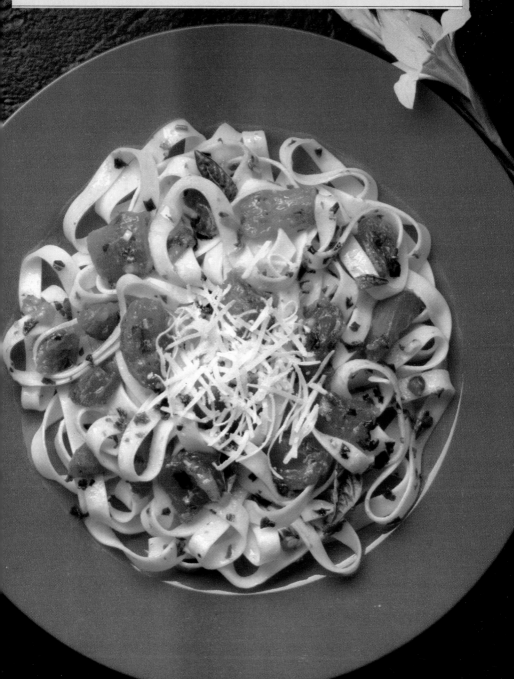

Pasta continues to grow in popularity because of its versatility and universal appeal. Sophisticated or simple—pasta is good for you. It is rich in carbohydrates and protein and low in sodium and cholesterol—until you add cheese, cream, butter or salt. Whole wheat pasta is more nutritious and flavorful than egg pasta which also contains cholesterol. The addition of vegetable purées to pasta dough enhances the taste, but only improves the nutritional content minimally. Pasta must cook quickly and constantly in rapidly boiling water. Cooking time varies with the different shapes and sizes, but regardless of shape or size it should be cooked just to the point that it is tender, yet still firm to the teeth. Don't rinse the pasta or you will have a loss of minerals and vitamins.

Rice is the staple food of over half the people in the world and provides a major source of protein. Rice is a good source of vitamins and minerals as well. Brown rice has a slightly nutty flavor and a chewier texture than white rice does and is a good source of dietary fiber.

Cuisines of the world are filled with celebrated dishes based on dried beans. Beans provide an excellent source of low-fat protein, carbohydrates and fiber. Lentils have been shown to help reduce cholesterol. They are inexpensive and give you top nutritional value for your dollar. Chick peas (garbanzo beans) and soybeans are higher in fat than other beans. (For instance, tofu, made from soybeans, is 43% fat.)

Recipe for this photograph on page 91.

BROCCOLI-NOODLE CASSEROLE

1 tablespoon corn oil margarine
2 tablespoons vegetable broth,
  either homemade or canned
2 cups fresh broccoli, chopped
1 pound fresh mushrooms,
  chopped
1 cup onion, chopped
¼ cup white wine
½ teaspoon salt (optional)
½ teaspoon pepper
3 eggs *
3 cups low-fat cottage cheese
1 cup low-fat plain yogurt
2 cloves garlic
2 teaspoons fresh basil or
  1 teaspoon dried basil
8 ounces whole wheat or
  white noodles
¼ cup bread crumbs
2 ounces low-fat Cheddar
  cheese, shredded

Preheat oven to 350 degrees. In a large skillet heat margarine and vegetable broth over medium heat. Sauté broccoli, mushrooms and onion in margarine and broth for 10 minutes. Mix in wine, salt and pepper; remove from heat. In a large bowl beat eggs with wire whisk. Mix in cottage cheese, yogurt, garlic and basil. Cook noodles according to package directions just until tender; drain well. In a large bowl place noodles. Add egg mixture; toss to mix. Add sautéed vegetables; mix well. Spray a 9x13-inch baking dish with vegetable cooking spray. Spoon in noodle mixture. Sprinkle with bread crumbs and Cheddar cheese; cover. Bake for 30 minutes; uncover. Bake for 15 minutes longer. Broccoli may be a combination of florets and peeled and sliced stems. Makes 8 servings.

* To reduce fat and cholesterol, use an egg substitute with less than 2 grams fat per serving.

Fat and calorie content may vary between brands.

Approx. per serving: 273.0 calories; 8.4 gr. fat; 27.69% calories from fat.

BROCCOLI-STUFFED SHELLS

An unusual variation of stuffed shells, this recipe can be made ahead of time and reheated before serving.

3 cups broccoli florets
1 container (15 ounces) part-skim
  ricotta cheese
1 egg * plus 2 egg whites
2 tablespoons Parmesan cheese,
  grated
1 teaspoon fresh oregano or
  ½ teaspoon dried oregano
½ teaspoon nutmeg
¼ teaspoon black pepper
24 jumbo pasta shells, cooked
1 cup Marinara Sauce
  (see page 72)

Preheat oven to 350 degrees. In a saucepan or steamer over medium heat cook broccoli until tender-crisp; drain and cool. In a food processor fitted with steel blade or using a sharp knife mince broccoli. In a bowl combine broccoli, ricotta cheese, egg and egg whites, Parmesan cheese, oregano, nutmeg and pepper; mix well. Into each pasta shell stuff about 1 tablespoon broccoli mixture. Into a baking dish pour Marinara Sauce. Arrange pasta shells in a single layer in prepared dish. Bake for 30 minutes. Makes 8 servings.

* To reduce fat and cholesterol, use an egg substitute with less than 2 grams fat per serving. Fat and calorie content may vary between brands.

Approx. per serving: 235.0 calories; 6.2 gr. fat; 23.74% calories from fat.

BULGUR WHEAT, PEPPERS AND TOFU

Tofu or bean curd (made from soy beans) is such a powerhouse of protein that the Chinese call it "meat without bones." It has a bland and creamy, nut-like flavor and can be cubed, cut into strips or crumbled depending on the recipe. It can be found in the supermarket produce department. Whole wheat kernels that are first steamed, dried and then crushed are called "bulgur." The combination of these two nutritious foods along with strips of pepper and spinach makes a splendid and colorful casserole.

1 cup bulgur wheat
1 tablespoon corn oil margarine
3 cloves garlic, minced
2 red bell peppers, cut into
  julienne strips
1 teaspoon cumin, ground
3 tablespoons cider vinegar
1 pound tofu (bean curd), cubed
10 ounces fresh spinach,
  washed, stemmed and
  coarsely chopped
1 teaspoon salt (optional)
½ teaspoon pepper, freshly ground

In a small bowl combine bulgur and enough cold water to cover. Let stand for 45 minutes or until tender. Into a fine sieve place bulgur. Press to remove as much moisture as possible. In a large skillet over medium heat melt margarine. Add garlic. Sauté for 30 seconds. Stir in red peppers and cumin; cover. Cook for 5 minutes. Add vinegar and bulgur. Cook, uncovered, for 5 minutes, stirring constantly. Add tofu and spinach; cover. Simmer for 5 minutes or until spinach wilts. Season with salt and pepper.
Makes 4 servings.

Approx. per serving: 288.0 calories; 8.6 gr. fat; 26.87% calories from fat.

CAPELLINI WITH CLAM SAUCE

Our version of an Italian clam sauce is made with sweet red peppers to add color and taste. The fresh parsley adds a garden-fresh flavor.

2 tablespoons corn oil margarine,
  divided
2 red bell peppers, cored, seeded
  and cut into thin strips
3 cloves garlic, minced, divided
Salt and freshly ground pepper
  to taste
1 dozen fresh shucked clams or
  1 can (5 ounces) clams, drained
1 cup dry white wine
1 teaspoon fresh thyme or
  ¼ teaspoon dried thyme
½ cup fresh parsley, minced
½ pound fresh or dried capellini
1½ tablespoons Parmesan
  cheese, grated

In a heavy skillet over medium heat melt 1 tablespoon margarine. Add peppers and ⅓ of the garlic. Sauté for 10 minutes or until peppers are tender. Season with salt and pepper. In a saucepan over medium heat melt the remaining 1 tablespoon margarine. Add the remaining garlic. Sauté for 1 minute. Add clams, wine and thyme. Simmer for 5 minutes. Add parsley and salt and pepper to taste. In a large pan of boiling water cook capellini *al dente*; drain. In warm oven heat dinner plates. Onto warm dinner plates spoon capellini. Top with clam sauce; arrange sautéed pepper strips around capellini. Sprinkle with Parmesan cheese.
Makes 3 main-course or 6 appetizer servings.

Approx. per serving: 406.0 calories; 10.5 gr. fat; 23.27% calories from fat.

FETTUCCINE WITH FRESH TOMATOES AND BASIL

This is a delightful supper in late summer or fall when tomatoes are at their best. For the most fiber, try whole wheat noodles.

6 ounces fettuccine
1 tablespoon olive oil
4 tomatoes, diced
2 cloves garlic, minced
2 teaspoons fresh basil, chopped
or ½ teaspoon dried basil
Pinch of granulated sugar
¼ cup fresh parsley, chopped
Salt and freshly ground pepper
to taste
2 tablespoons Parmesan cheese, grated

In a large pan of boiling salted water cook fettuccine *al dente*; drain. In a heavy skillet heat oil over medium heat. Add tomatoes, garlic, basil and sugar. Cook for 5 minutes, stirring occasionally. Add parsley, salt and pepper. Add to tomato mixture with cheese; toss to mix. Makes 2 main-course or 4 appetizer or side-dish servings.

Approx. per serving: 545.0 calories; 13.2 gr. fat; 21.79% calories from fat; high fiber.

Photograph for this recipe on page 87.

LINGUINI WITH TOMATO, BASIL, SPINACH AND CAPERS

Italians like to have fun with the names for their pasta. "Linguini" means tongues, "fettuccine" means narrow ribbons and "capelli" means angel hair. This sauce is so good, you can serve it over any pasta shape you choose.

2 pounds tomatoes, peeled, seeded and coarsely chopped
1 cup fresh basil, coarsely chopped
2 tablespoons olive oil, divided
⅓ cup onion, finely chopped
⅓ cup carrot, finely chopped
⅓ cup celery, finely chopped
2 cloves garlic, crushed
1 jar (3¼ ounces) capers, drained and rinsed
2 tablespoons vinegar
Salt and pepper to taste
1 pound spinach or whole wheat linguini

In a bowl mix tomatoes and basil; set aside. In a skillet heat 1 tablespoon olive oil over low heat. Add onion. Sauté just until translucent. Add carrot, celery and garlic. Sauté for 1 minute. Add tomato mixture. Simmer, uncovered, for 20 minutes. Add capers, vinegar and salt and pepper. In a large pan of boiling water cook linguini *al dente*; drain. Add the remaining 1 tablespoon oil to the linguini; toss to coat. Onto a large serving platter place linguini. Top with tomato sauce. Makes 6 servings.

Approx. per serving: 194.0 calories; 5.6 gr. fat; 25.97% calories from fat.

CHEESE AND SPINACH MANICOTTI

Although a number of ingredients and several different steps are involved in making manicotti, it is not a difficult dish to make. Be sure to drain pasta well before stuffing.

8 manicotti shells
1½ cups part-skim ricotta cheese
1 egg*
1 package (10 ounces) frozen chopped spinach, thawed and squeezed dry
¼ cup Parmesan cheese, freshly grated, divided
1 teaspoon fresh basil or ½ teaspoon dried basil
1 clove garlic, minced
½ teaspoon salt (optional)
½ teaspoon pepper
⅛ teaspoon nutmeg
4 cups Marinara Sauce, (see page 72), divided

Preheat oven to 375 degrees. Cook manicotti shells according to package directions. In a bowl combine ricotta cheese, egg, spinach, 2 tablespoons Parmesan cheese, basil, garlic, salt, pepper and nutmeg; mix well. Stuff into manicotti shells. Into a 9x13-inch baking dish pour 1 cup Marinara Sauce. Arrange stuffed shells in single layer in prepared dish. Mix any remaining filling with remaining 3 cups Marinara Sauce. Pour over manicotti. Sprinkle with remaining 2 tablespoons Parmesan cheese. Cover pan with foil. Bake for 1 hour. Makes 8 manicotti.

* To reduce fat and cholesterol, use an egg substitute with less than 2 grams fat per serving. Fat and calorie content may vary between brands.

Approx. per manicotti: 261.0 calories; 10.4 gr. fat; 35.86% calories from fat; high vitamin A.

COLD PASTA PRIMAVERA

"Primavera" means spring in Italian. This delicate pasta dish was created by a chef in New York City to utilize the bounty of spring vegetables. Almost any vegetable can be used. Try snow peas, asparagus, string beans or zucchini.

2 ounces whole wheat or white small shell or bow tie pasta
1 cup broccoli florets, chopped
1 cup fresh peas or frozen peas, thawed and drained
1 cup red or green bell pepper, thinly sliced
1 cup tomatoes, chopped
½ cup fresh parsley, chopped
2 scallions, sliced
2 tablespoons low-fat cottage cheese
1 or 2 tablespoons 1% low-fat milk
¼ cup low-fat plain yogurt
1 teaspoon fresh oregano or ½ teaspoon dried oregano
1 teaspoon fresh basil or ½ teaspoon dried basil
½ teaspoon salt (optional)
¼ teaspoon pepper
¼ cup Parmesan cheese, freshly grated

Cook pasta according to package directions; drain and cool. In separate saucepans over medium heat cook broccoli and peas in a small amount of water just until tender-crisp; drain and cool. In a medium bowl combine pasta, broccoli, peas, bell pepper, tomatoes, parsley and scallions; toss to mix. In a blender container combine cottage cheese and milk; process until smooth. In a small bowl combine blended cottage cheese, yogurt, oregano, basil, salt and pepper; blend well. Add to pasta, tossing to coat. Add Parmesan cheese; toss gently until well coated. Chill in refrigerator. Serve chilled. Makes 4 servings.

Approx. per serving: 170.0 calories; 3.4 gr. fat; 18.0% calories from fat; high fiber.

PASTA WITH PEPPERS AND PARMESAN

2 tablespoons corn oil margarine
2 tablespoons olive oil
2 red or green bell peppers, quartered and thinly sliced
1 clove garlic, minced
½ teaspoon salt (optional)
¼ teaspoon pepper
8 ounces whole wheat or white fettuccine or other flat pasta
3 tablespoons Parmesan cheese, freshly grated

In a large skillet combine margarine and olive oil. Heat over low heat until margarine melts. Add bell peppers and garlic. Sauté for 5 minutes. Add salt and pepper. Sauté for 2 minutes. Keep warm. Cook fettuccine *al dente* using package directions; drain. In a serving bowl combine hot fettuccine, sautéed pepper and cheese; toss to mix. Serve at once. Makes 6 servings.

Approx. per servings: 204.0 calories; 3.4 gr. fat; 15.0% calories from fat.

CREAMY PASTA WITH BROCCOLI

1 small bunch broccoli, cut into florets
1 small head cauliflower, cut into florets
2½ cups whole wheat or egg noodles
1 tablespoon olive oil or corn oil
3 cloves garlic, minced
2½ cups fresh mushrooms, thickly sliced
1 cup low-fat small-curd cottage cheese
¼ cup 1% low-fat milk
¼ cup Parmesan cheese, grated
Salt and cayenne pepper to taste

In a large pan of boiling, salted water cook broccoli and cauliflower for 5 minutes or until tender-crisp. With a slotted spoon remove vegetables; reserve cooking liquid. Bring reserved liquid to a boil over medium-high heat. Add pasta. Cook for 8 to 10 minutes or *al dente*; drain. In a large skillet heat oil over medium heat. Add garlic. Sauté for 2 minutes. Add mushrooms. Sauté for 5 minutes. Add broccoli and cauliflower. Sauté for 2 to 3 minutes longer. In a food processor combine cottage cheese, milk and Parmesan cheese. Process until smooth. Add to broccoli mixture with pasta; toss to mix. Season with salt and cayenne pepper. Serve immediately. Makes 8 servings.

Approx. per serving: 220.0 calories; 4.9 gr. fat; 20.04% calories from fat; high fiber.

SLIM
SPAGHETTI PIE

4 ounces vermicelli
3 tablespoons Parmesan cheese, grated
1 egg, * well beaten
¾ pound ground chuck
⅔ cup onion, chopped
¼ cup green pepper, chopped
1 can (8 ounces) stewed tomatoes
1 can (6 ounces) tomato paste
1½ teaspoons fresh oregano or
¾ teaspoon dried whole oregano
1 clove garlic, minced or
½ teaspoon garlic salt
½ cup low-fat cottage cheese
¼ cup part-skim mozzarella cheese, shredded
2 teaspoons fresh parsley, chopped

Cook vermicelli according to package directions, omitting salt; drain. In a large bowl add Parmesan cheese to hot vermicelli; stir until well mixed. Add egg; mix well. Spray 9-inch glass pie plate with vegetable cooking spray. Into the prepared pie plate spoon vermicelli; press over bottom and side, forming pie shell. Microwave, uncovered, on High for 2 minutes or until set. Set aside. In a shallow 2-quart casserole crumble ground beef; stir in onion and green pepper. Cover with heavy duty plastic wrap. Microwave on High for 5 minutes, stirring every 2 minutes. Into a colander place ground beef mixture; drain. Pat dry with paper towels. Wipe the casserole with the paper towels. In the casserole combine drained ground beef mixture, tomatoes, tomato paste, oregano and garlic; mix well. Cover with plastic wrap. Microwave on High for 3½ minutes, stirring once. Layer cottage cheese and ground beef sauce in prepared pie plate. Cover with plastic wrap. Microwave on High for 6 minutes.

Uncover. Sprinkle with mozzarella cheese. Microwave on High for 30 seconds or until cheese begins to melt. Sprinkle with parsley. Let stand for 10 minutes before serving. Makes 6 servings.

* To reduce fat and cholesterol, use an egg substitute with less than 2 grams fat per serving. Fat and calorie content may vary between brands.

Approx. per serving: 267.0 calories; 10.6 gr. fat; 35.73% calories from fat.

LEAN
QUESIDILLAS

Quesidillas look like small Mexican pizzas. They make a nutritious meal in a hurry.

6 corn tortillas
3 ounces part-skim mozzarella cheese, shredded
Lettuce, shredded
1½ cups alfalfa sprouts
Tomato slices or chunks
1 cup Mock Sour Cream (see page 84)
Green Salsa (see page 80)

In an ungreased hot skillet toast tortillas on both sides. Top with cheese. Heat until cheese melts. Place tortillas on serving plate. Layer lettuce, alfalfa sprouts, tomato slices and Mock Sour Cream. Serve with salsa. Makes 6 servings.

Approx. per serving: 141.0 calories; 4.2 gr. fat; 26.8% calories from fat.

VEGETARIAN LASAGNA

12 whole wheat or white
lasagna noodles, divided
1 cup part-skim ricotta cheese
1 cup low-fat cottage cheese
½ cup fresh parsley,
finely chopped
2 cloves garlic, minced
¼ teaspoon nutmeg
Pepper to taste
4 cups Marinara Sauce
(see page 72), divided
½ pound part-skim mozzarella
cheese, grated, divided
2 tablespoons Parmesan cheese,
freshly grated

Preheat oven to 375 degrees. Cook lasagna noodles *al dente* using package directions; drain. In a small bowl combine ricotta cheese, cottage cheese, parsley, garlic, nutmeg and pepper; mix well. In a 9x13-inch baking dish spread 1 cup Marinara Sauce. Arrange 4 noodles over sauce. Spoon half the cottage cheese mixture over noodles in small mounds 2 inches apart. Spoon 1 cup sauce over cottage cheese mixture. Sprinkle with half the mozzarella cheese. Repeat layers with 4 noodles, the remaining cottage cheese mixture, 1 cup sauce and the remaining mozzarella cheese. Layer the remaining 4 noodles and 1 cup sauce on top. Sprinkle with Parmesan cheese. Cover. Bake for 35 minutes. Uncover. Bake for 10 minutes longer. Let stand for 5 to 10 minutes before serving. Makes 8 servings.

Approx. per serving: 335.0 calories; 13.2 gr. fat; 35.46% calories from fat.

SPAGHETTI WITH SPINACH AND MUSHROOMS

½ pound fresh mushrooms,
trimmed and thinly sliced
1 tablespoon fresh lemon juice
Corn oil margarine
2 tablespoons Madeira
2 cloves garlic, minced
1 cup 1% low-fat milk
½ teaspoon salt (optional)
¼ teaspoon pepper
1 package (10 ounces) frozen
chopped spinach, thawed
and drained
½ pound whole wheat or
white spaghetti
2 tablespoons Parmesan cheese,
freshly grated

In a small bowl combine mushrooms and lemon juice. In a large skillet over low heat melt margarine. Add Madeira and garlic. Cook for 3 minutes. Add mushrooms. Cook for 5 minutes. Add milk, salt and pepper. Bring to a boil over medium heat, stirring constantly. Drain spinach well. To the mushroom mixture add spinach. Simmer for 5 minutes. Remove from heat; keep warm. Cook spaghetti *al dente* using package directions; drain. In a serving dish combine spinach mixture and hot spaghetti; toss to combine well. Sprinkle each serving with ½ tablespoon Parmesan cheese. Makes 4 servings.

Approx. per serving: 257.0 calories; 4.8 gr. fat; 16.8% calories from fat; high vitamin A.

GARDEN
CHILI

Serve this chili with Elegant Rice Ring (see page 98) for an impressive main dish. This recipe makes approximately 5 quarts so freeze some for a quick meal after a busy day at work.

**3 tablespoons corn oil or
safflower oil
3 large onions, chopped
3 zucchini, sliced
1 pound fresh mushrooms,
chopped
2 or 3 leeks, thoroughly cleaned
and chopped
1 clove garlic, minced
2 tablespoons chili powder
2 teaspoons mustard seed
1 teaspoon cumin seed
¼ teaspoon cardamom, ground
¼ teaspoon cinnamon
2 cans (20 ounces each)
tomatoes
1 can (16 ounces) stewed
tomatoes
1 can (6 ounces) tomato paste
1 cup beer or water
1 tablespoon vinegar
1 tablespoon light brown sugar
3 cans (16 ounces each)
kidney beans
Part-skim mozzarella cheese,
shredded
Low-fat plain yogurt
Green onions, chopped
Salsa (see page 80)
Tomatoes, chopped
Lettuce, shredded
Tortilla chips, slightly crushed
Green chilies, chopped**

In a large kettle heat oil over low heat. Add onions, zucchini, mushrooms, leeks, garlic, chili powder, mustard seed, cumin seed, cardamom and cinnamon. Sauté for several minutes. Cut canned tomatoes into large chunks. To the sautéed vegetables add tomatoes, tomato paste, beer, vinegar and brown sugar. Add beans. Cook over low heat for 45 to 60 minutes or until thickened.

Into soup bowls ladle chili. Into individual serving bowls place cheese, yogurt, green onions, salsa, tomatoes, lettuce, tortilla chips and chilies. Garnish chili with desired toppings. Makes 10 to 12 servings.

Approx. per serving: 262.0 calories; 5.6 gr. fat; 19.23% calories from fat; high fiber.

VERMICELLI
WITH BROCCOLI

**1 bunch fresh broccoli
2 tablespoons corn oil margarine
3 scallions, sliced
1 clove garlic, minced
2 tablespoons white wine
1 teaspoon fresh lemon juice
½ teaspoon salt (optional)
¾ pound whole wheat vermicelli
1 tablespoon olive oil
¼ cup Parmesan cheese,
freshly grated**

Cut broccoli into florets; peel and slice stems. In a saucepan or steamer steam broccoli florets and stems in a small amount of water until tender-crisp. Into a colander place broccoli. Rinse gently with cold water; drain. In a medium skillet over medium heat melt margarine. Add scallions and garlic. Sauté for 2 minutes. Add wine. Cook for 5 minutes. Add broccoli, lemon juice and salt. Cook until heated through. Cook vermicelli *al dente* using package directions; drain. In a serving bowl combine hot vermicelli and olive oil; toss to coat. Add broccoli mixture; toss gently. Sprinkle with Parmesan cheese. Serve immediately. Makes 8 servings.

Approx. per serving: 259.0 calories; 6.7 gr. fat; 23.28% calories from fat.

BAKED RICE

While roasting chicken, assemble the ingredients for this baked rice dish and cook for the last 20 minutes of the chicken roasting time. If oven space is needed for other dishes, the rice can be simmered on the range for 20 minutes.

2 cups chicken broth, either
   homemade or canned
1 tablespoon corn oil margarine
2 scallions, sliced
¼ teaspoon salt (optional)
¼ teaspoon pepper
1 cup uncooked white rice
¾ cup fresh parsley, chopped

Preheat oven to 375 degrees. In a saucepan over medium-high heat bring chicken broth to a boil; cover. Set aside to keep warm. In an ovenproof skillet over medium-high heat melt margarine. Add scallions. Sauté until tender. Add salt and pepper. Reduce heat to medium. Add rice. Sauté for 5 minutes. Stir in hot broth carefully. Add parsley; cover. Place on center oven rack. Bake for 20 minutes or until liquid is absorbed. Fluff with a fork before serving.
Makes 4 servings.

Approx. per serving: 240.0 calories; 6.74 gr. fat; 25.27% calories from fat.

BRAZILIAN RICE

A vegetable rice medley is an excellent accompaniment to meat entrées, or it can make a tasty main dish on its own.

3 tablespoons olive oil, divided
½ pound fresh mushrooms, sliced
½ cup onion, chopped
½ cup cabbage, finely chopped
1 clove garlic, minced
1 can (6 ounces) tomato paste
⅓ cup water
1 teaspoon fresh basil or
  ½ teaspoon dried basil
½ teaspoon salt (optional)
¼ teaspoon pepper
⅛ teaspoon celery seed
1½ cups uncooked brown rice
3 cups hot water

In a medium skillet heat 1½ tablespoons olive oil over low heat. Add mushrooms, onion, cabbage and garlic. Sauté for 10 minutes. Add tomato paste, ⅓ cup water, basil, salt, pepper and celery seed; mix well. Simmer, covered, for 20 minutes. In a large skillet heat the remaining 1½ tablespoons olive oil. Add rice. Sauté until light brown. Add 3 cups hot water. Simmer, covered, for 30 minutes. Stir in vegetable mixture. Simmer, covered, for 10 minutes longer or until rice is tender.
Makes 8 servings.

Approx. per serving: 195.0 calories; 4.4 gr. fat; 20.3% calories from fat.

BROWN RICE PILAF

Brown rice contains slightly more fiber than white rice while adding a crunchier texture.

½ cup uncooked brown rice
⅓ cup onion, chopped
⅓ cup fresh mushrooms, sliced
¼ teaspoon pepper
¼ teaspoon fresh thyme or
   ⅛ teaspoon dried thyme
1¼ cups chicken broth, either
   homemade or canned
½ cup celery, thinly sliced

Preheat oven to 350 degrees. In a 1-quart casserole combine rice, onion, mushrooms, pepper and thyme. Stir in broth; cover. Bake for 1 hour. Add celery; mix well. Cover. Bake for 10 to 15 minutes or until celery is just tender and liquid is absorbed.
Makes 4 servings.

Approx. per serving: 107.0 calories; 1.0 gr. fat; 8.4% calories from fat.

ELEGANT RICE RING

Unmold this rice ring on a heated serving plate and fill the center with Garden Chili (see page 96) or with an Oriental-style main dish.

4 cups chicken broth, either
   homemade or canned
2 cups uncooked rice
1 tablespoon corn oil margarine
4 stalks celery, sliced diagonally
½ large onion, minced
1 package (10 ounces) frozen
   tiny peas, cooked and drained
3 tablespoons fresh parsley,
   chopped
Parsley sprigs

In a large saucepan bring chicken broth to a boil. Stir in rice; cover and reduce heat. Simmer for 20 minutes or until rice is tender. In a skillet over low heat melt margarine. Add celery and onion. Sauté until tender. Stir sautéed vegetables, peas and chopped parsley into rice. Into a ring mold press rice mixture. Onto a serving plate invert rice ring. Garnish with parsley sprigs. Serve immediately.
Makes 8 servings.

Approx. per serving: 235.0 calories; 2.5 gr. fat; 9.57% calories from fat.

HARVEST RICE

This unusual rice dish is an excellent accompaniment to roast turkey or chicken.

**1 tablespoon corn oil margarine
1 cup carrots, thinly sliced
1¼ cups water
¾ cup apple juice
2 tablespoons fresh lemon juice
2 tablespoons light brown sugar
1 teaspoon salt (optional)
1 cup rice
½ cup raisins
½ teaspoon cinnamon
2 cups unpeeled apples, sliced
½ cup green onions, sliced
1 tablespoon sesame seed, toasted**

In a large skillet over low heat melt margarine. Add carrots. Sauté for 5 minutes or until tender-crisp. Add water, apple and lemon juice, brown sugar and salt; mix well. Bring to a boil over medium heat. Stir in rice, raisins and cinnamon; cover and reduce heat. Simmer for 15 minutes or until rice is tender. Stir in apples and green onions. Cook until heated through. Into a serving dish spoon rice mixture. Sprinkle sesame seed over top. Makes 6 servings.

Approx. per serving: 246.0 calories; 3.1 gr. fat; 11.34% calories from fat; high vitamin A.

LEMON PILAF

**1 teaspoon corn oil margarine
⅓ cup celery, sliced
⅓ cup green onions with tops, sliced
1 cup cooked rice
1 teaspoon lemon rind, grated
¼ teaspoon salt (optional)
Dash of pepper**

In a skillet over low heat melt margarine. Add celery and green onions. Sauté until tender. Add rice, lemon rind, salt and pepper. Heat to serving temperature, stirring occasionally.
Makes 2 servings.

Approx. per serving: 134.0 calories; 1.9 gr. fat; 12.76% calories from fat.

MEATLESS CABBAGE ROLLS

An easy and fast way to cook cabbage leaves is to use your microwave oven. Separate leaves and arrange in a casserole dish. Sprinkle with water, cover and microwave on High for 6 minutes.

1 head cabbage
1 tablespoon corn oil margarine
1 cup carrots, chopped
1 cup onion, chopped
1½ cups cooked brown rice
2 cups broth, either homemade or canned
1 tablespoon fresh lemon juice
½ teaspoon salt (optional)
¼ teaspoon each pepper, cumin and celery seed
6 ounces part-skim mozzarella cheese, shredded
1 can (28 ounces) tomatoes, coarsely chopped
2 tablespoons cornstarch
2 tablespoons water

Preheat oven to 375 degrees. Remove core from cabbage, leaving head intact. In a large saucepan place cabbage head; cover with boiling water. Cover saucepan partially. Cook over medium heat for 10 minutes. Remove cabbage carefully; drain. Remove 16 to 20 outer leaves; pat dry and set aside. In a large skillet over low heat melt margarine. Sauté carrots and onion for 5 minutes. Stir in rice, ½ cup broth, lemon juice, salt, pepper, cumin and celery seed; cover. Simmer for 15 minutes. Remove from heat; cool slightly. Stir in cheese. Trim thick center vein from each cabbage leaf. Place 3 to 4 tablespoons filling in center; roll to enclose filling, folding in sides. Secure with toothpick or thread. In a 9 x 13-inch baking dish arrange cabbage rolls seam side down. Pour tomatoes with juice and the remaining 1½ cups broth over cabbage rolls; cover. Bake for 1 hour; uncover. Bake for 30 minutes longer, basting frequently. On a serving platter place cabbage rolls. In a small saucepan pour pan juices. Bring to a boil over medium heat. In a small bowl blend cornstarch with 2 tablespoons cold water. Stir into boiling liquid. Cook until thickened, stirring constantly. Serve over cabbage rolls. Makes 8 servings.

Approx. per serving: 165.0 calories; 5.9 gr. fat; 32.18% calories from fat; high vitamin A; high fiber.

SPANISH RICE

1 pound lean ground beef or ground chuck
1 cup uncooked rice
1 mild onion, chopped
1 green bell pepper, chopped
1 slice garlic
4 cups canned tomatoes
1 tablespoon chili powder
1 teaspoon salt (optional)
¼ teaspoon fresh marjoram or ⅛ teaspoon dried marjoram (optional)

Preheat oven to 350 degrees. In a skillet over medium heat brown ground beef, stirring until crumbly; drain thoroughly, reserving pan drippings. Into a 3-quart casserole place ground beef. In the skillet sauté rice in reserved pan drippings until brown. Add onion, green pepper and garlic. Sauté for 5 minutes longer. Add tomatoes, chili powder, salt and marjoram; mix well. Cook until heated through. Stir into ground beef in casserole; cover. Bake for 45 minutes. Makes 6 to 8 servings.

Approx. per serving: 304.0 calories; 10.2 gr. fat; 30.19% calories from fat.

TURKISH TOMATOES AND RICE

2 tablespoons olive oil
4 large onions, thinly sliced
2 pounds tomatoes, cut into halves
¼ cup uncooked rice
1 teaspoon granulated sugar
1 teaspoon cumin
Salt and pepper to taste
1 cup water
Juice of ½ lemon
2 tablespoons fresh parsley, chopped

In a skillet heat olive oil over low heat. Add onions. Sauté for 5 to 6 minutes. In a saucepan arrange tomato halves in a single layer. Layer sautéed onions and rice over tomatoes. Sprinkle with sugar, cumin, salt and pepper. Add water and lemon juice; cover. Cook over medium heat for 15 minutes or until tomatoes and rice are tender. Into a serving dish place tomatoes and rice. Sprinkle with parsley. Serve warm or at room temperature. Makes 6 to 8 servings.

Approx. per serving: 140.0 calories; 5.1 gr. fat; 32.78% calories from fat; high fiber.

NORTHWOODS WILD RICE AND BRUSSELS SPROUTS

Wild rice is not actually rice, but the seed of a water grass grown at the edges of the lakes in the northern United States. For many years it was harvested by Chippewa Indians, but it is now being commercially cultivated. It has a strong, nut-like flavor and a chewy texture.

7 or 8 Brussels sprouts, washed and trimmed
3 tablespoons corn oil margarine
2 tablespoons green onion, chopped
1 clove garlic, minced
3 cups cooked wild rice
Salt and pepper to taste

In a saucepan cook Brussels sprouts in boiling water to cover for 12 minutes or until tender. Drain and coarsely chop. In a heavy saucepan over low heat melt margarine. Add green onion and garlic. Sauté until tender but not brown. Add chopped Brussels sprouts; mix well. Add wild rice; toss gently. Into a heated serving dish spoon rice mixture. Add salt and pepper. Makes 6 to 8 servings.

Approx. per serving: 177.0 calories; 6.4 gr. fat; 32.54% calories from fat.

BLACK BEANS AND RICE

Black beans can be served over rice or as a thick hearty soup.

1 pound dried black beans, washed and drained
6 cups water
2 bay leaves
½ teaspoon salt (optional)
¼ teaspoon pepper
4 ounces lean ham or turkey ham, chopped
2 tablespoons olive oil
1 cup onion, chopped
1 green bell pepper, chopped
1 clove garlic, crushed
4 cups hot cooked rice
8 fresh sweet onion rings

In a large saucepan place beans and enough water to cover. Bring to a boil over medium-high heat. Boil for 2 minutes; remove from heat. Cover. Let stand for 1 hour; drain. To the beans add 6 cups water, bay leaves, salt and pepper. Stir in ham. Bring to a boil over medium heat. Reduce heat; cover. Simmer for 2 hours, adding additional water if necessary. Remove bay leaves. In a small skillet heat olive oil over low heat. Add onion, green pepper and garlic. Sauté for several minutes. To the bean mixture add sautéed vegetables. Into individual serving bowls spoon rice. Spoon beans over rice. Top each serving with an onion ring. Makes 8 servings.

Approx. per serving: 341.0 calories; 5.0 gr. fat; 13.19% calories from fat; high fiber.

HOPPIN' JUAN

Mexican-inspired Hoppin' Juan can become a complete meal with heated tortillas and a fresh green salad.

1½ cups uncooked brown rice
½ cup dried black-eyed peas, cooked
1 large onion, chopped
3 fresh jalapeño peppers or 1 can (8 ounces) jalapeño peppers, finely chopped
3 cloves garlic, minced
Salt to taste
4 cups part-skim mozzarella cheese, shredded, divided
½ pound part-skim ricotta cheese
2 tablespoons 1% low-fat milk

Cook brown rice according to package directions. Preheat oven to 350 degrees. In a large bowl combine rice, black-eyed peas, onion, jalapeño peppers, garlic and salt; mix well. In a medium bowl combine 3 cups mozzarella cheese, ricotta cheese and milk; mix well. In a large casserole layer rice mixture and ricotta mixture alternately until all ingredients are used, ending with rice mixture. Bake for 25 minutes. Sprinkle with remaining 1 cup mozzarella cheese. Bake for 5 minutes longer. Makes 12 servings.

Approx. per serving: 170.0 calories; 7.9 gr. fat; 41.82% calories from fat.

FRESH AND HEALTHY TOSTADA

Tostadas are Mexican open-faced sandwiches. Try tomatoes and lettuce instead of zucchini and spinach.

2 corn tortillas
½ cup Lentils Olé
   (see following recipe)
½ cup fresh spinach, chopped
¼ cup carrot, shredded
¼ zucchini, unpeeled, shredded
¼ to ½ cup low-fat plain yogurt
Mock Sour Cream (see page 84)
Salsa (see page 80)
2 tablespoons sunflower seed

In an ungreased heavy skillet place tortillas 1 at a time. Warm over medium-high heat for 15 seconds on each side. On a serving plate place tortillas. Layer lentils, spinach, carrot, zucchini, yogurt, Mock Sour Cream, a generous drizzle of salsa and sunflower seed. Makes 1 serving. Nutritional information does not include Mock Sour Cream.

Approx. per serving: 359.0 calories; 12.3 gr. fat; 30.83% calories from fat; high vitamin A; high fiber.

LENTILS OLÉ

The nutritious legume that we call lentils starts as a dry bean-like pellet and becomes a delicious earthy treat. Our spicy Mexican version is delicious on or with tacos, enchiladas, tostados or burritos.

3 cups water
1 cup lentils
1 tablespoon corn oil or
   safflower oil
½ cup green onions and tops,
   chopped
½ cup green bell pepper,
   chopped
4 cloves garlic, minced
1 tablespoon chili powder
½ teaspoon cumin seed, crushed
1 can (8 ounces) tomato sauce
1 tablespoon red wine vinegar
1 tablespoon molasses

In a large saucepan combine water and lentils. Bring to a boil over medium-high heat. Cover. Reduce heat to medium-low. Simmer for 20 to 30 minutes or until lentils are tender but firm. Set aside. In a medium skillet heat oil over low heat. Add green onions, green pepper, garlic, chili powder and cumin seed. Stir-fry for 2 minutes or until vegetables are tender-crisp. Stir in tomato sauce, vinegar and molasses. Simmer for 1 minute. Into lentils stir tomato mixture. Cook until heated through. Makes 3 cups (½ cup per serving).

Approx. per serving: 149.0 calories; 2.6 gr. fat; 15.7% calories from fat.

LENTIL STEW

Parsley and carrots are great sources of vitamin A in this well-flavored lentil stew.

3½ cups chicken broth, either
   homemade or canned
1 can (16 ounces) whole
   tomatoes, undrained and
   coarsely chopped
2 large onions, chopped
1 cup lentils
2 medium carrots, scraped
   and chopped
½ cup fresh parsley, chopped
¼ cup dry Sherry
½ teaspoon dried whole thyme
½ teaspoon dried whole marjoram
½ teaspoon pepper

In a stockpot combine broth, tomatoes, onions, lentils, carrots, parsley, Sherry, thyme, marjoram and pepper. Bring to a boil over medium-high heat. Cover. Reduce heat to medium-low. Simmer for 45 minutes or until lentils are tender. Makes 8½ cups.

Approx. per cup: 132.0 calories; 0.85 gr. fat; 5.79% calories from fat; high vitamin A; high fiber.

RED BEANS AND RICE

¾ pound ham hocks, washed
1 quart water
1 pound dried red beans,
   sorted and washed
1½ cups onions, chopped
1 cup fresh parsley, chopped
1 cup green bell pepper, chopped
1 can (8 ounces) tomato sauce
½ cup green onions, chopped
1 clove garlic, pressed
1 tablespoon Worcestershire
   sauce
1 teaspoon black pepper
½ teaspoon red pepper
½ teaspoon fresh oregano or
   ¼ teaspoon dried oregano
½ teaspoon fresh thyme or
   ¼ teaspoon dried thyme
3 dashes of hot sauce
5 cups hot cooked rice

In a large saucepan place ham hocks and water. Bring to a boil over medium-high heat; cover. Reduce heat to medium-low. Simmer for 30 minutes or until tender. Remove and discard ham hocks. Strain broth. Chill overnight. Remove surface fat. Set broth aside. Into a stockpot place beans and water to cover. Let stand overnight. Drain. Add ham broth. Cover. Cook over low heat for 45 minutes. Add onions, parsley, green pepper, tomato sauce, green onions, garlic, Worcestershire sauce, black and red peppers, oregano, thyme and hot sauce. Cover. Cook over low heat for 2 to 2½ hours, stirring occasionally and adding additional water if desired. Serve over rice. Makes 10 servings. A ½ cup serving of rice adds 90 calories.

Approx. per serving: 192.0 calories; 0.96 gr. fat; 4.5% calories from fat.

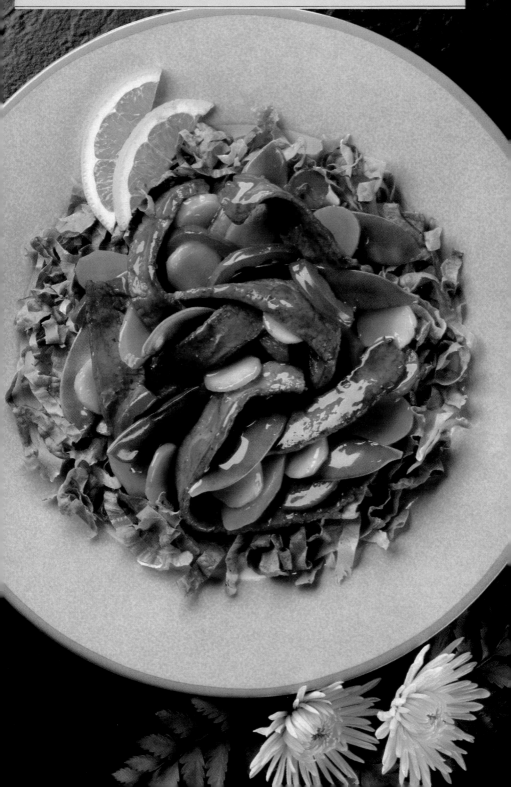

The following poultry, seafood and meat recipes are nutritionally balanced, energy boosting and delicious. It's perfectly possible to enjoy full-flavored, satisfying meals that are relatively low in calories, fat and salt but high in vitamins and fiber.

The versatility and economy of poultry can't be beat. Except for special occasions, avoid fatty poultry, as duck or goose. Turkey meat or the meat from small chickens is the most lean. While some are broth-basted, most self-basting birds are basted with butter or fat, such as coconut oil, which adds cholesterol. Always remove the skin from chicken before cooking it.

Lean veal can have as little as one-tenth the fat of lean beef. Buy only the leanest cuts of red meat, and trim off all visible fat. Serve small sensible portions. The U.S. Dietary Guidelines recommend four ounces of meat, poultry or fish as a portion. Always broil or roast meats and poultry on a rack or broiling pan so that the fat can drip off.

Fish allows you to create marvelous meals for a healthier diet. Fish can be poached, steamed, baked, grilled, broiled or cooked in the microwave. Don't overcook fish. The best guide is the 10-Minute Rule: For each inch of thickness, cook for 10 minutes. Test the fish with a fork at its thickest point; if the fish is opaque, it is done. Four ounces of broiled steak has 30 to 45 grams of fat, which is largely saturated. The same amount of broiled fish contains 4 to 8 grams of mostly polyunsaturated fat. The fat in the steak accounts for about 70% of the meat's total caloric content while fat represents only 35% of the total calories in fish.

Recipe for this photograph on page 107.

GINGER-ORANGE BEEF

This easy-to-make Chinese delight will please your family and guests. Serve it with rice. If the flank steak is slightly frozen, you will be able to slice it neatly and easily.

3 pounds flank steak
1 tablespoon corn oil or safflower oil
¼ cup fresh gingerroot, freshly grated
3 cups carrots, diagonally sliced
3 cups red bell peppers, chopped
3 cups green bell peppers, chopped
2 cups water chestnuts, sliced
8 ounces fresh snow peas, trimmed
2 tablespoons orange rind, grated
1 tablespoon cinnamon
⅓ cup lite soy sauce
1 tablespoon cornstarch
2 heads iceberg lettuce, shredded

Slice steak into ¼-inch thick strips. In a large skillet or wok heat oil over medium heat. Add gingerroot. Stir-fry for 1 minute. Add steak. Stir-fry for 3 minutes or until steak is cooked through. Remove steak; keep warm. Add carrots. Stir-fry for 1 minute. Add red and green peppers, water chestnuts, snow peas, orange rind and cinnamon. Stir-fry for 3 minutes or until vegetables are tender-crisp. Add steak. In a small bowl mix soy sauce and cornstarch. Stir into steak and vegetable mixture. Cook until thickened, stirring constantly. Onto serving plate place lettuce. Spoon steak mixture onto lettuce. Makes 12 servings.

Approx. per serving: 235.0 calories; 6.9 gr. fat; 26.42% calories from fat; high vitamin A; high fiber.

Photograph for this recipe on page 105.

FRENCH BEEF STEW WITH VEGETABLES

This hearty dish is fine for a mid-winter meal. When the lid of the casserole is lifted, an aroma sweeps across the table that will tempt any appetite. You can make this stew several days ahead since the flavor only improves with time. Make a double batch and freeze half for when there is no time to cook.

2 pounds boneless beef roast, all fat removed
8 medium potatoes, quartered
8 medium carrots, quartered
1 large onion, sliced
2 cloves garlic, minced
1 teaspoon fresh thyme or ½ teaspoon dried thyme
½ teaspoon salt (optional)
¼ teaspoon pepper
½ cup red wine
2 tablespoons corn oil margarine, softened
2 tablespoons all-purpose flour
1 cup fresh parsley, chopped

Preheat oven to 250 degrees. In a Dutch oven place roast. Arrange potatoes, carrots and onion around and over roast. Sprinkle with garlic, thyme, salt and pepper; drizzle wine over top. Cover. Roast for 4½ hours. On a serving platter place roast; slice if desired. Surround with the vegetables. Keep warm. Place the Dutch oven with pan juices over high heat. Cook until bubbly. In a small bowl blend margarine and flour into a smooth paste; stir into the pan juices. Cook until thickened, whisking constantly. Spoon a small amount over roast and vegetables; sprinkle with parsley. Into a gravy boat pour remaining gravy. Serve with roast. Makes 8 (3-ounce) servings.

Approx. per serving: 339.0 calories; 11.4 gr. fat; 30.26% calories from fat; high vitamin A.

PEPPER STEAK

1 tablespoon corn oil or
  safflower oil
1 pound round steak,
  cut into strips
3 medium tomatoes, peeled,
  seeded and cored
2 green bell peppers,
  cut into strips
1 cup fresh mushrooms, sliced
1 medium onion, sliced
2 tablespoons lite soy sauce
1 teaspoon salt (optional)
½ teaspoon ginger
½ teaspoon granulated sugar
¼ teaspoon pepper
2 tablespoons all-purpose flour

In a large skillet heat oil over medium heat. Add steak. Sauté until brown. Add tomatoes, green peppers, mushrooms and onion. Stir in soy sauce, salt, ginger, sugar and pepper; cover. Simmer for 30 minutes. In a small bowl blend a small amount of pan juices with flour. Stir into skillet. Cook until thickened, stirring constantly. Serve over rice. Makes 6 servings.

Approx. per serving: 196.0 calories; 8.3 gr. fat; 38.11% calories from fat.

PORTUGUESE CABBAGE ROLLS

This recipe recalls country cooking— familiar, comforting ingredients combined in a homey manner. The cabbage may be cooked in a micro- wave oven (see page 100 for Meatless Cabbage Rolls).

1 head cabbage
1 tablespoon corn oil margarine
1 tablespoon broth, either
  homemade or canned,
  fat removed
1 cup carrots, grated
1 cup onion, chopped
1 pound lean ground round
2 cups cooked brown rice
1 tablespoon fresh lemon juice
1 teaspoon fresh oregano or
  ½ teaspoon dried oregano
1 teaspoon fresh thyme or
  ½ teaspoon dried thyme
½ teaspoon salt (optional)
¼ teaspoon pepper
1 can (28 ounces) tomatoes,
  drained and coarsely chopped
2 cups beef broth, either
  homemade or canned

Preheat oven to 375 degrees. Remove core from cabbage, leaving head intact. Into a large pan of boiling water place cabbage head. Cover loosely. Cook for 10 minutes. Lift out carefully; drain. Remove 16 to 20 outer leaves; pat dry. In a skillet over medium heat melt margarine with broth. Add carrots and onion. Sauté over medium-high heat for 5 minutes. Add ground round, rice, lemon juice, oregano, thyme, salt and pepper. Cook for 10 minutes or until ground round is brown and crumbly, stirring frequently. Trim thick center ribs from cabbage leaves. Onto each leaf spoon 3 to 4 tablespoons ground round mix- ture. Roll cabbage leaf to enclose filling, tucking in ends; secure with thread or toothpicks. In a 9 x 13-inch baking pan arrange cabbage rolls. In a bowl mix to- matoes and beef broth. Pour over rolls; cover. Bake for 1 hour. Un- cover. Bake for 30 minutes longer, basting frequently. If rolls begin to brown, cover with foil. (For thicker sauce pour sauce into saucepan. Bring to a boil over medium heat. In a small bowl blend 2 table- spoons cornstarch in 2 tablespoons water. Stir into sauce. Cook until thickened, whisking constantly.) Makes 8 servings.

Approx. per serving: 227.0 calories; 9.2 gr. fat; 36.47% calories from fat; high vitamin A; high fiber.

SOUTH AMERICAN CHILI BEEF IN TORTILLAS

A great new recipe for chili lovers everywhere—a colorful blend of green peppers, tomato sauce and tender beef. For added "fire" include a jalapeño pepper, seeded and finely chopped.

1 tablespoon corn oil or
   safflower oil
1 cup onion, chopped
2 cloves garlic, minced
2 pounds beef round, cut into
   small cubes, all fat removed
2 tablespoons all-purpose flour
1 cup green bell pepper, chopped
1 cup tomato sauce
3 tablespoons canned mild
   green chilies, chopped
2 tablespoons red wine vinegar
2 teaspoons fresh oregano or
   1 teaspoon dried oregano
1 teaspoon cumin, ground
½ teaspoon salt (optional)
10 large whole wheat or
   white flour tortillas
2½ cups lettuce, shredded

In a large saucepan heat oil over medium heat. Add onion and garlic. Sauté until tender. Add beef. Sauté over medium-high heat for 5 minutes. Add flour; toss with beef cubes until coated. Add green pepper, tomato sauce, green chilies, vinegar, oregano, cumin and salt; mix well. Cover. Simmer over medium heat for 2½ hours, stirring every 30 minutes. Uncover. Simmer for 30 minutes longer or until slightly thickened. Heat tortillas according to package directions until warm but not crisp. Onto each tortilla spoon beef mixture. Add ¼ cup lettuce to each; roll to enclose filling. Makes 10 servings.

Approx. per serving: 264.0 calories; 7.5 gr. fat; 25.56% calories from fat.

STEW ALLA SICILIANA

Make a habit of trimming fat from meat before cooking. You'll never miss the empty calories.

2 pounds lean stew beef
1 can (16 ounces) tomatoes
1 cup beef broth, either
   homemade or canned
½ cup dry red wine
¼ cup tapioca
3 cloves garlic, minced
3 bay leaves
2 teaspoons each fresh marjoram,
   oregano and basil or 1 teaspoon
   each dried
1 teaspoon salt (optional)
1 teaspoon granulated sugar
1 teaspoon fresh thyme or
   ½ teaspoon dried thyme
½ teaspoon black pepper
½ teaspoon dry red pepper
   flakes (optional)
2 medium onions, cut into chunks
4 stalks celery, cut into chunks
2 to 4 medium potatoes,
   cut into chunks
4 to 6 carrots, cut into chunks
½ pound fresh mushrooms
1 package (10 ounces) frozen
   peas, thawed

Preheat oven to 275 degrees. In a 6-quart Dutch oven combine beef, tomatoes, broth, wine and tapioca; mix well. Add garlic, bay leaves, marjoram, oregano, basil, salt, sugar, thyme, black pepper and red pepper flakes; mix well. Stir in onions and celery; cover. Bake for 4 hours. Add potatoes and carrots; cover. Bake for 1¼ hours or until vegetables are tender. In a skillet over medium heat sauté mushrooms. Stir mushrooms and peas into stew. Bake or cook over low heat for 15 minutes longer. Discard bay leaves. Makes 6 to 8 servings.

Approx. per serving: 500.0 calories; 16.3 gr. fat; 29.34% calories from fat; high fiber.

STUFFED SHELLS WITH BEEF AND TOMATO SAUCE

*For a taste of Italy try this excep-
tionally good filling stuffed into
pasta shells. The dish may be
assembled the day before and
baked just before serving.*

18 jumbo pasta shells
½ pound lean ground chuck
1 small onion, chopped
Cloves garlic to taste, minced
1 can (15 ounces) tomato sauce
1 can (6 ounces) tomato paste
1½ teaspoons fresh oregano or
¾ teaspoon dried oregano
½ teaspoon pepper
1½ cups low-fat cottage cheese
3 tablespoons Parmesan cheese,
grated
1 egg,* beaten
2 tablespoons fresh parsley,
minced
Dash of nutmeg

Preheat oven to 350 degrees.
Cook pasta shells according to
package directions, omitting salt;
drain and set aside. Spray a large
skillet with vegetable cooking
spray. Over medium heat place
skillet; add ground chuck, onion
and garlic. Cook until brown and
crumbly, stirring frequently. Into
colander place mixture; drain well
then pat dry with paper towels.
With fresh paper towels wipe skillet. Into skillet place ground chuck
mixture. Add tomato sauce, tomato paste, oregano and pepper;
mix well. Bring to a boil over
medium heat; reduce heat. Simmer, uncovered, for 15 minutes. In
a medium bowl combine cottage
cheese, Parmesan cheese, egg,
parsley and nutmeg; mix well.
Into each pasta shell stuff 1
rounded tablespoon cottage cheese
mixture. Into an 8x12-inch baking
dish spoon sauce. Arrange shells
in prepared dish; cover. Bake for
40 minutes. Makes 6 servings.

* To reduce fat and cholesterol,
use an egg substitute with less
than 2 grams fat per serving.
Fat and calorie content may vary
between brands.

*Approx. per serving: 325.0 calories;
10.1 gr. fat; 27.96% calories from fat.*

STUFFED PEPPERS CALIFORNIA

1 pound lean ground round
1½ cups cooked brown rice
1 egg,* beaten
½ cup carrots, grated
2 teaspoons fresh oregano or
1 teaspoon dried oregano
½ teaspoon salt (optional)
½ teaspoon pepper
8 medium green bell peppers
2 cups fresh tomatoes, chopped
1 cup tomato sauce
½ cup onion, finely chopped
1 tablespoon fresh lemon juice

Preheat oven to 350 degrees. In
a bowl combine ground round,
rice, egg, carrots, oregano, salt
and pepper; mix well. Cut peppers
into halves lengthwise; remove
membrane and seed. Spoon mixture into pepper shells. Into a large
baking dish place stuffed peppers;
do not crowd. In a medium bowl
combine tomatoes, tomato sauce,
onion and lemon juice; mix well.
Spoon over and around peppers.
Cover with foil. Bake for 1 hour.
Serve immediately.
Makes 8 servings.

* To reduce fat and cholesterol,
use an egg substitute with less
than 2 grams fat per serving.
Fat and calorie content may vary
between brands.

*Approx. per serving: 203.0 calories;
8.4 gr. fat; 37.24% calories from fat.*

CHINESE BEEF
STIR-FRY

1 pound flank steak, fat trimmed
½ cup water
¼ cup lite soy sauce
1 tablespoon cornstarch
1½ teaspoons granulated sugar
1 medium onion
3 stalks celery, diagonally sliced
½ pound fresh mushrooms, sliced
½ cup water chestnuts, sliced
½ pound fresh snow peas
3 cups hot cooked rice

Partially freeze steak. Slice cross grain into ¼x2-inch strips; set aside. In a small bowl combine water, soy sauce, cornstarch and sugar; set aside. Peel onion, slice ¼ inch thick and cut each slice into quarters; set aside. Spray a wok with vegetable cooking spray. Heat over medium-high heat for 2 minutes. Add steak to wok. Stir-fry for 3 minutes. With a slotted spoon remove steak; set aside. Add onion, celery, mushrooms and water chestnuts to wok. Stir-fry for 2 to 3 minutes. Add steak and snow peas; cover. Reduce heat to medium. Simmer for 2 to 3 minutes. Stir in soy sauce mixture. Cook over medium-high heat until thickened and bubbly, stirring constantly. Serve over rice. Makes 6 servings.

Approx. per serving: 277.0 calories; 3.9 gr. fat; 12.67% calories from fat.

CHINESE PORK
AND VEGETABLES

1 tablespoon corn oil or
   safflower oil
1 pound lean boneless pork,
   cut into thin strips
5 stalks celery, diagonally sliced
4 carrots, diagonally sliced
1 medium onion, sliced
1 tablespoon fresh gingerroot,
   grated
2 cloves garlic, minced
1 cup hot broth, either
   homemade or canned
2 tablespoons lite soy sauce
¼ teaspoon pepper, freshly ground
1 small head cabbage
2 tablespoons cold water
1 tablespoon cornstarch
Fresh lemon juice to taste
Salt and freshly ground pepper
   to taste

In a wok or large heavy skillet heat oil over high heat. Add pork. Stir-fry until pork is no longer pink. Add celery, carrots, onion, gingerroot and garlic. Stir-fry until onion is tender. Add broth, soy sauce and ¼ teaspoon pepper; cover. Simmer for 5 minutes. Shred cabbage; measure 4 cups packed cabbage. Stir into wok. Cook for 3 to 4 minutes or until vegetables are tender-crisp. In a small bowl mix cold water and cornstarch. Stir into wok. Cook until thickened, stirring constantly. Add lemon juice, salt and pepper to taste. Makes 5 servings.

Approx. per serving: 352.0 calories; 13.6 gr. fat; 34.77% calories from fat; high vitamin A.

VENETIAN LIVER

The liver should be cut to an even thickness of ¼ inch. The thinner the liver is, the faster it cooks, and the sweeter it tastes. It should be a pale, rosy color.

**1 tablespoon olive oil
1 cup onion, thinly sliced
1 clove garlic, minced
¼ teaspoon fresh sage or
    ⅛ teaspoon dried sage
1 pound calves liver, sliced
    into ¼-inch strips
½ teaspoon salt (optional)
½ teaspoon pepper
¼ cup white wine
¼ cup fresh parsley, chopped
6 cups hot cooked brown rice**

In a heavy skillet heat oil over medium heat. Add onion, garlic and sage. Sauté for 10 minutes. With a slotted spoon remove onion; set aside. With paper towels pat liver slices dry; sprinkle with salt and pepper. To the hot skillet add liver. Cook for 2 to 3 minutes or until liver is no longer red. Return sautéed onion to skillet; mix lightly. With a slotted spoon remove liver and onion; set aside. Add wine to skillet. Bring to a boil over medium heat. Boil for 2 minutes, stirring to deglaze skillet. Return liver and onion to skillet; spoon sauce over liver. Heat to serving temperature. Sprinkle with parsley. Serve over brown rice. Makes 5 servings.

Approx. per serving: 446.0 calories; 7.0 gr. fat; 14.12% calories from fat; high vitamin A; high fiber.

CHICKEN AND DUMPLINGS

**1 (2½ to 3-pound) chicken,
    skinned
1 teaspoon salt (optional)
2 cups self-rising flour
1 egg,* slightly beaten**

In a 4-quart saucepan place chicken with water to cover; cover. Cook over medium heat until tender. Remove chicken; bone and cut into bite-sized pieces. Chill broth until fat congeals on top; remove fat. In a bowl combine flour, ¾ cup broth and egg; mix well. On a floured board roll out dough. Cut into strips. In the saucepan bring remaining broth to a boil over medium heat. Add dumplings. Cook for 5 minutes. Add chicken. Cook for 10 minutes. Makes 4 servings.

* To reduce fat and cholesterol, use an egg substitute with less than 2 grams fat per serving. Fat and calorie content may vary between brands.

Approx. per serving: 708.0 calories; 12.0 gr. fat; 15.25 % calories from fat.

CHICKEN CACCIATORE

A perennial on the menu of Italian restaurants, Chicken Cacciatore or Hunter's Chicken is a classic dish that is worth the little extra time and attention it requires. Don't economize on the quality of the wine—a wine not good enough to drink is not good enough to use in cooking.

2 tablespoons olive oil
3 tablespoons corn oil margarine, divided
3 pounds chicken pieces, skinned
½ pound mushrooms, sliced
2 medium green peppers, chopped
1 medium onion, chopped
2 cloves garlic, minced
1 can (6 ounces) tomato paste
½ cup dry white wine
¼ cup parsley or 2 tablespoons dried parsley
1½ teaspoons salt (optional)
½ teaspoon fresh oregano or ¼ teaspoon dried oregano
½ teaspoon fresh thyme or ¼ teaspoon dried thyme
½ cup water
8 ounces vermicelli

In a skillet heat olive oil and 2 tablespoons margarine. Add chicken. Cook over medium-high heat until brown. Remove chicken; reserve 2 tablespoons pan drippings. To the drippings add mushrooms, green peppers, onion and garlic. Stir-fry until onion is tender. Add tomato paste, wine, parsley, salt, oregano and thyme. Stir in water. Arrange chicken over vegetables. Simmer for 45 minutes, stirring occasionally. Cook vermicelli using package directions; drain. In a deep serving dish combine hot vermicelli and remaining 1 tablespoon margarine; toss to coat. On the vermicelli arrange chicken. Spoon sauce over chicken. Makes 4 to 5 servings.

Approx. per serving: 932.0 calories; 26.4 gr. fat; 25.49% calories from fat.

CHICKEN FRIED RICE

1 tablespoon corn oil or safflower oil
½ cup carrots, grated
1 cup cooked chicken, chopped
2 eggs,* lightly beaten
½ teaspoon pepper
3 cups cooked brown rice
3 tablespoons lite soy sauce
⅔ cup scallions, sliced

In a wok or skillet heat oil over medium heat. Add carrots and chicken. Stir-fry for 1 minute. Add eggs and pepper. Stir-fry for 1 minute. Add rice and soy sauce. Stir-fry for 5 minutes. Garnish with scallions. Serve immediately. Makes 6 servings.

* To reduce fat and cholesterol, use an egg substitute with less than 2 grams fat per serving. Fat and calorie content may vary between brands.

Approx. per serving: 202.0 calories; 5.4 gr. fat; 24.05% calories from fat.

CHICKEN WITH PASTA AND SNOW PEAS

Pasta combines well with thousands of flavors and textures—including Oriental ingredients such as fresh ginger and snow peas.

1 pound tomato rotelle (corkscrew pasta)
1 chicken, skinned, boned and boiled, poached or baked
4 ounces Chinese snow peas
1 bunch green onions, finely chopped
1 slice (1 inch) fresh gingerroot, grated
¼ to ½ cup red wine vinegar
3 tablespoons extra virgin olive oil
Salt and pepper to taste

Cook rotelle using package directions for 8 minutes or until *al dente*. Rinse with cold water; drain. Shred chicken. In a saucepan over medium-high heat blanch snow peas in a small amount of boiling water. Into a bowl of ice water place snow peas; drain. Combine rotelle, chicken, snow peas, green onions and gingerroot in bowl. In a small bowl combine vinegar, olive oil, salt and pepper; mix well. Pour over rotelle; mix gently. Garnish with additional snow peas.
Makes 4 to 6 servings.

Approx. per serving: 565.0 calories; 14.8 gr. fat; 23.57% calories from fat.

CRISPY HERBED CHICKEN

6 chicken pieces (2 pounds), skinned
½ cup all-purpose flour
4 teaspoons fresh basil or 2 teaspoons dried basil
4 teaspoons fresh thyme or 2 teaspoons dried thyme
2 teaspoons salt (optional)
2 teaspoons fresh oregano or 1 teaspoon dried oregano
2 teaspoons fresh tarragon or 1 teaspoon dried tarragon
1 teaspoon paprika
½ teaspoon pepper
⅓ cup warm water

Preheat oven to 375 degrees. Rinse chicken under cold running water; pat dry. In a lightly greased shallow roasting pan place chicken in a single layer. In a small jar combine flour, basil, thyme, salt, oregano, tarragon, paprika and pepper. Cover and shake well. Sprinkle 2 tablespoons herb-seasoned flour mixture on chicken. Store remaining herb-seasoned flour in the covered jar at room temperature. Pour warm water down side of pan; do not pour on chicken. Bake for 40 to 50 minutes or until tender, basting with pan juices occasionally.
Makes 6 servings.

Approx. per serving: 257.0 calories; 5.4 gr. fat; 18.91% calories from fat.

HERB-BAKED CHICKEN

1 (3-pound) broiler-fryer, skinned
  and cut up
2 teaspoons fresh rosemary or
  1 teaspoon dried rosemary
Pepper to taste
½ cup unsweetened pineapple
  juice
¼ teaspoon ginger, ground
5 shallots, minced
Paprika

Preheat oven to 350 degrees. Rub chicken with rosemary and pepper. In a 9-inch baking dish arrange chicken pieces meaty sides up. In a bowl combine pineapple juice and ginger. Pour over chicken. Sprinkle with shallots and paprika; cover. Bake for 30 minutes. Uncover. Bake for 25 to 30 minutes or until tender. Makes 6 servings.

Approx. per serving: 325.0 calories; 6.8 gr. fat; 18.83% calories from fat.

LO-CAL CHICKEN STEW

1 (3 to 3½-pound) chicken,
  skinned and cut up
8 medium potatoes, cut into
  eighths
2 large onions, cut into eighths
1 large green bell pepper,
  cut into strips
Sliced carrots
Salt and pepper to taste

Spray a skillet with vegetable cooking spray. In the prepared skillet over medium-high heat brown chicken. Add potatoes, onions, green pepper, carrots, salt and pepper. Simmer for 45 minutes or until chicken is tender. Makes 5 servings.

Approx. per serving: 676.0 calories; 10.2 gr. fat; 13.57% calories from fat; high Vitamin A; high fiber.

MICROWAVE PINEAPPLE CHICKEN

Microwaved chicken is moist and tender. Besides being quick and easy, use of the Brown-in-Bag means there is no messy clean-up.

1 (3-pound) chicken, skinned and cut up
Salt and pepper to taste
1 Brown-in-Bag
1 medium onion, sliced
½ medium green bell pepper, cut into strips
2 cans (8 ounces each) tomato sauce
1 tablespoon cornstarch
1 can (8 ounces) crushed pineapple, drained
1 tablespoon light brown sugar
2 teaspoons fresh lemon juice
½ teaspoon salt (optional)
¼ teaspoon ginger

Sprinkle chicken with salt and pepper to taste. In a glass 2-quart baking dish place Brown-in-Bag. In the Brown-in-Bag arrange chicken with larger pieces around edges. Place onion and green pepper over chicken. In a small bowl blend tomato sauce and cornstarch. Stir in pineapple, brown sugar, lemon juice, ½ teaspoon salt and ginger; mix well. Pour over chicken. Close bag tightly; do not use twist-tie with metal strip. Make six ½-inch slits in bag. Microwave on High for 28 to 30 minutes or until chicken is tender, turning dish once. Makes 4 servings.

Approx. per serving: 558.0 calories; 10.5 gr. fat; 16.93% calories from fat.

ORANGE CHICKEN

For a wonderful supper, serve this slightly sweet chicken with rice or pasta and a garden salad.

1 chicken, skinned and cut up
Salt and pepper to taste
All-purpose flour
2 tablespoons corn oil or safflower oil
1 large onion, sliced
1 can (6 ounces) frozen orange juice concentrate

Preheat oven to 350 degrees. Sprinkle chicken with salt and pepper. Coat with flour. In a large skillet heat oil over medium heat. Add chicken. Cook over medium-high heat until brown. In a 9x13-inch baking dish arrange chicken. In the skillet sauté onion in the pan drippings until tender. Spoon onion over chicken. Spread orange juice concentrate over chicken. Bake for 1 hour. Serve with rice. Makes 4 servings.

Approx. per serving: 656.0 calories; 17.0 gr. fat; 23.32% calories from fat.

PARMESAN-YOGURT CHICKEN

Yogurt acts as a tenderizer making chicken succulent and delectable.

1 (2-pound) fryer, skinned and
    cut up
2 tablespoons fresh lemon juice
Salt and black pepper to taste
½ cup low-fat plain yogurt
¼ cup lite mayonnaise
¼ cup scallions, sliced
2 tablespoons Dijon mustard
1 tablespoon Worcestershire
    sauce
1 teaspoon fresh thyme or
    ½ teaspoon dried thyme
¼ teaspoon cayenne pepper
¼ cup Parmesan cheese,
    freshly grated

Preheat oven to 350 degrees. In a large glass baking dish arrange chicken in a single layer. Drizzle with lemon juice. Sprinkle with salt and pepper. In a small bowl combine yogurt, mayonnaise, scallions, mustard, Worcestershire sauce, thyme and cayenne pepper; mix well. Spread over chicken. Bake for 50 minutes. Drain off juices. Preheat broiler. Sprinkle cheese over chicken. Broil chicken 4 inches from heat source for about 3 minutes or until cheese melts and browns slightly.
Makes 4 to 6 servings.

Approx. per serving: 424.0 calories; 9.0 gr. fat; 19.10% calories from fat.

SAUTÉED CHICKEN WITH YOGURT AND MUSHROOMS

6 chicken pieces, skinned
1 tablespoon all-purpose flour
2 teaspoons corn oil margarine
2 medium onions, thinly sliced
¼ pound fresh mushrooms, sliced
½ cup water (or ¼ cup water and
    ¼ cup white wine)
½ cup low-fat plain yogurt
Salt and freshly ground pepper
    to taste

Sprinkle chicken pieces with flour. In a large nonstick skillet melt margarine over medium-high heat. Add chicken. Cook for 5 minutes on each side or until brown. Reduce heat to medium. Cook for 10 minutes on each side or until cooked through. In a warm oven heat a baking dish. Place chicken on warm dish; keep warm. Add onions and mushrooms to the skillet. Cook for 5 to 10 minutes or until tender, stirring frequently. Stir in water. Bring to a full rolling boil over high heat, stirring to deglaze skillet. Remove from heat. Stir in yogurt, salt and pepper. Arrange chicken pieces in skillet; spoon sauce over top.
Makes 6 servings.

Approx. per serving: 302.0 calories; 7.2 gr. fat; 21.45% calories from fat.

SUPER CHICKEN

2 fryers, skinned and cut up
1 tablespoon seasoned salt
(optional)
1 cup chicken bouillon
¼ cup dry white wine
2 teaspoons fresh onion, chopped
or ½ teaspoon instant onion
½ teaspoon curry powder
¼ cup water
2 tablespoons all-purpose flour
1 cup fresh mushrooms or 1 can
(4 ounces) mushrooms, sliced

Preheat oven to 350 degrees. Sprinkle chicken with seasoned salt. In a baking dish arrange chicken pieces. In a small bowl combine bouillon, wine, onion and curry powder; mix well. Pour over chicken. Cover with foil. Bake for 30 minutes. Uncover. Bake for 30 minutes longer or until chicken is tender. Into a strainer over a small saucepan pour pan juices. In a small bowl blend water and flour. Add to pan juices. Cook over low heat until thickened, stirring constantly. Add mushrooms. Heat to serving temperature. On a serving plate arrange chicken. Spoon gravy over chicken. Makes 6 servings.

Approx. per serving: 650.0 calories; 13.8 gr. fat; 19.10% calories from fat.

CHICKEN-APPLE SAUTÉ

1 tablespoon corn oil or
safflower oil
1 pound chicken breasts, skinned,
boned and cut into strips
1 cup celery, diagonally sliced
1 medium green bell pepper,
sliced lengthwise
1 medium onion, sliced lengthwise
1 Golden Delicious apple, cored
and sliced
½ cup apple juice
1 tablespoon white wine vinegar
1 tablespoon cornstarch
1 teaspoon lite soy sauce

In a wok or nonstick skillet heat oil over medium heat. Add chicken. Sauté over medium-high heat until cooked through. Remove chicken. Add celery, green pepper and onion. Stir-fry until tender-crisp. Add chicken and apple. Stir-fry for 1 minute. In a small bowl combine apple juice, vinegar, cornstarch and soy sauce. Add to chicken. Cook until thickened, stirring constantly.
Makes 4 servings.

Approx. per serving: 238.0 calories; 6.9 gr. fat; 26.09% calories from fat.

CHICKEN FAJITAS

From the East to the West Coast, Tex-Mex cooking is sweeping the country. These piquant tidbits of chicken provide an easy introduction to this exciting food fad. For variety top with Red Salsa and a dollop of Mock Sour Cream (see page 84).

**2 pounds boneless chicken
    breasts, skinned and cut into
    ¾-inch strips
⅓ cup dry Sherry
¼ cup olive oil
3 jalapeño peppers, seeded and
    finely chopped
1 tablespoon chili powder
2 teaspoons cumin, ground
1 medium clove garlic,
    finely chopped
Shredded lettuce**

In a shallow dish place chicken. In a small bowl combine Sherry, olive oil, peppers, chili powder, cumin and garlic; mix well. Pour over chicken. Marinate at room temperature for 2 hours or in refrigerator overnight, stirring occasionally. Preheat broiler. Drain chicken, reserving marinade. In a broiling pan arrange chicken. Broil 3 inches from heat source for 3 to 4 minutes on each side, basting occasionally with marinade. Serve with fresh corn tortillas and Green Salsa (see page 80). Top with lettuce. Makes 6 servings.

Approx. per serving: 352.0 calories; 14.6 gr. fat; 37.32% calories from fat.

CHICKEN PAPRIKA

We usually use paprika to dust on salads or fish for a little color, but it is a seasoning that has long given gusto to Hungarian cooking. And, it is Hungary that produces the finest paprika. Store paprika in a cool, dark place to keep it fresh.

**1 ½ tablespoons corn oil or
    safflower oil
2 whole chicken breasts,
    skinned, boned and cut into
    1½-inch pieces
1 cup fresh mushrooms, sliced
½ cup onion, chopped
½ cup chicken broth, either
    homemade or canned
1 tablespoon paprika
1 teaspoon fresh dill or
    ½ teaspoon dried dillweed
¼ teaspoon pepper
2½ cups uncooked egg noodles
2 tablespoons cold water
1 tablespoon cornstarch
1 cup low-fat plain yogurt**

In a large skillet heat oil over medium heat. Add chicken, mushrooms and onion. Sauté over medium-high heat until tender. Add broth, paprika, dill and pepper; cover. Reduce heat. Simmer for 10 minutes or until chicken is tender. Cook noodles according to package directions using unsalted water; drain. In a small bowl blend water and cornstarch. Stir into chicken mixture. Cook for 1 minute, stirring constantly. Remove from heat. Stir in yogurt. Serve over noodles. Makes 4 servings.

Approx. per serving: 486.0 calories; 10.4 gr. fat; 19.25% calories from fat.

CHICKEN AND FRESH VEGETABLE SAUTÉ

1 tablespoon corn oil margarine
4 chicken breast halves,
   skinned and boned
1 or 2 medium tomatoes, wedged
1 medium onion, wedged
1 medium zucchini, cut into strips
¼ teaspoon pepper, freshly ground

In a large skillet over medium heat melt margarine. Add chicken. Cook over medium-high heat for 10 to 12 minutes or until brown on both sides. Add tomato, onion and zucchini. Sprinkle with pepper; cover. Reduce heat. Cook over low heat for 5 to 7 minutes or until vegetables are tender-crisp. Makes 4 servings.

Approx. per serving: 193.0 calories; 6.1 gr. fat; 28.44% calories from fat.

CHICKEN WITH GRAPES AND MUSHROOMS

This extravagantly delicious combination lends itself beautifully to entertaining. It's the perfect dish for the buffet table. For the freshest taste choose mushrooms with tightly closed caps.

1 tablespoon unbleached flour
¼ teaspoon salt (optional)
¼ teaspoon pepper
2 pounds boneless chicken
   breasts, skinned and cut into
   bite-sized pieces
2 tablespoons corn oil margarine
¼ cup onion, minced
½ pound small fresh mushrooms
¾ cup chicken broth, either
   homemade or canned
½ cup white wine
½ cup 1% low-fat milk
1 tablespoon cornstarch
1 tablespoon water
1 cup seedless grapes

Preheat oven to 325 degrees. In a bag combine flour, salt and pepper. In the seasoned flour shake chicken to coat. In a skillet heat margarine over medium heat. Add chicken. Sauté until light brown. Into a casserole spoon chicken with slotted spoon. To the skillet add onion. Cook over low heat until onion is tender. Add mushrooms. Cook for 3 minutes. Spoon over chicken. To the skillet add broth and wine. Bring to a boil over medium heat. Add milk. Return to the boiling point. Simmer over medium-high heat for 5 minutes. In a small bowl blend cornstarch and water. Stir into simmering sauce. Cook until thickened, stirring constantly. Pour over chicken. Cover the casserole. Bake for 20 minutes. Add grapes. Bake for 10 minutes longer. Serve immediately. Makes 8 servings.

Approx. per serving: 211.0 calories; 6.4 gr. fat; 27.29% calories from fat.

CHICKEN PICCATTA CAPER

Capers are small, unopened flower buds from a Mediterranean bush that are pickled in vinegar. The tiny ones from the south of France are considered the finest. Their pungent flavor is a contrast to the mild chicken. Don't overcook the chicken breasts.

8 chicken breast halves, skinned and boned
½ cup all-purpose flour
Salt and pepper to taste
Paprika to taste
2 tablespoons corn oil margarine
1 tablespoon olive oil
2 to 4 tablespoons dry Madeira or Sherry
3 tablespoons fresh lemon juice
3 to 4 tablespoons capers

With a meat mallet or heavy plate flatten chicken breasts between sheets of waxed paper. In a bowl combine flour, salt, pepper and paprika. Coat chicken with seasoned flour; shake off excess. In a large skillet over medium heat melt margarine and olive oil. Add chicken. Sauté over medium-high heat for 2 to 3 minutes on each side. Remove chicken; drain on paper towel. To the skillet add Madeira, stirring to deglaze. Add lemon juice. Cook until heated through. Add chicken. Heat to serving temperature. On a heated serving plate arrange chicken. Garnish with capers.

Approx. per serving: 293.0 calories; 10.2 gr. fat; 31.33% calories from fat.

CHICKEN SCALOPPINE

Serve chicken alongside the cooked rice (start cooking rice about 20 minutes before beginning chicken recipe, so they will be done at the same time). Spoon some of the sauce over the rice.

2 tablespoons corn oil margarine
1 pound boneless chicken breasts, cut into thin "scaloppine" slices
¼ cup dry white wine
2 tablespoons chicken broth, either homemade or canned
1 tablespoon fresh lemon juice
2 teaspoons capers
2 cups hot cooked brown rice

In a skillet over medium heat melt margarine. Add chicken. Sauté over medium-high heat for 1 minute on each side. Remove chicken; keep warm. To the skillet add wine, broth and lemon juice. Bring to a boil over medium heat. Cook for 3 minutes, stirring to deglaze skillet. Add capers and chicken, turning chicken to coat with sauce. Reduce heat. Simmer for 5 minutes. Serve over rice. Makes 4 servings.

Approx. per serving: 320.0 calories; 9.4 gr. fat; 26.43% calories from fat.

CHICKEN SUKIYAKI

This opulent adaptation of the famous Japanese dish is equally good made with shrimp.

1 tablespoon corn oil or
  safflower oil
3 chicken breasts, skinned,
  boned and sliced
1 small onion, sliced
1 cup water chestnuts, sliced
⅔ cup celery, sliced diagonally
⅔ cup red bell pepper, sliced
  diagonally
1 cup bamboo shoots, sliced
  diagonally
⅔ cup fresh mushrooms, sliced
1 ½ cups fresh spinach
⅔ cup white wine
⅔ cup water
⅓ cup lite soy sauce
1 can (3 ounces) Chinese noodles

In a large nonstick skillet, cast iron skillet or wok heat oil over medium-high heat. Add chicken and onion. Stir-fry until chicken is cooked through. Heat a serving plate in warm oven. Spoon chicken mixture onto warm plate; keep warm. Add water chestnuts, celery, red pepper, bamboo shoots, mushrooms and spinach to skillet 1 at a time in order listed, stir-frying for several seconds after each addition. In a small bowl mix wine, water and soy sauce. Stir into vegetables. Add chicken mixture. Reduce heat to medium. Cook for 5 to 6 minutes. Onto a serving plate spoon sukiyaki. Serve over rice. Sprinkle with noodles. May use any vegetable of choice.
Makes 6 servings.

Approx. per serving: 285.0 calories; 9.1 gr. fat; 28.73% calories from fat.

CHICKEN TERIYAKI

"Teri" translates from the Japanese as "gloss" or "luster" and describes the sheen of the sauce that goes over the broiled (yaki) chicken, fish, beef or pork. You may want to make a double batch of sauce since it will keep indefinitely in the refrigerator in a sealed bottle.

6 chicken breast halves
  (8 ounces each), skinned
1 cup dry white wine
½ cup water
⅓ cup lite soy sauce
1 clove garlic, finely minced
½ teaspoon ginger, ground

In a large shallow dish place chicken breasts. In a small bowl combine wine, water, soy sauce, garlic and ginger; mix well. Pour over chicken; cover. Marinate in refrigerator overnight. Preheat broiler. Spray broiler rack with vegetable cooking spray; place in broiler pan. Drain chicken, reserving marinade. On the prepared broiler rack arrange chicken breasts. Broil 8 to 10 inches from heat source for 10 to 15 minutes on each side, basting occasionally with reserved marinade.
Makes 6 servings.

Approx. per serving: 343.0 calories; 6.7 gr. fat; 17.58% calories from fat.

CHICKEN-VEGETABLE STIR-FRY

6 chicken breast halves
   (8 ounces each), skinned, boned
   and cut into 1 ½-inch pieces
¼ cup plus 1 tablespoon
   lite soy sauce
2 small green bell peppers,
   cut into 1-inch strips
1 large onion, coarsely chopped
½ cup fresh mushrooms or 1 can
   (4 ounces) mushrooms, sliced
1 can (8 ounces) water chestnuts,
   drained and sliced
1 teaspoon cornstarch
¾ teaspoon granulated sugar
⅛ teaspoon red pepper
3 cups hot cooked rice

Spray wok or skillet with vegetable cooking spray. Heat over medium-high heat for 1 to 2 minutes. Add chicken and soy sauce. Stir-fry for 3 to 4 minutes or until light brown. Remove chicken from wok with slotted spoon. To the wok add green peppers and onion. Stir-fry for 4 minutes or until tender-crisp. Drain mushrooms, reserving any liquid. Add chicken, mushrooms and water chestnuts to stir-fried vegetables. In a small bowl combine the reserved mushroom liquid, cornstarch, sugar and red pepper; mix well. Stir into chicken mixture. Reduce heat. Simmer for 2 to 3 minutes or until slightly thickened, stirring constantly. Serve over rice. Makes 6 servings.

Approx. per serving: 469.0 calories; 7.0 gr. fat; 13.43% calories from fat.

FRUITED CHICKEN BREASTS

Chicken has always been a favorite entrée because it is delicious and inexpensive and lends itself to great variety in preparation. This recipe is sure to be a happy addition to your cooking repertory.

6 chicken breast halves, skinned
   and boned
1 tablespoon corn oil margarine
¼ teaspoon cardamom
¼ teaspoon salt (optional)
Dash of pepper
2½ to 3 cups firm baking apples,
   unpeeled and thinly sliced
⅓ cup cider
¼ cup granulated sugar
1 tablespoon fresh lemon juice
1 ½ teaspoons grated lemon rind
1 teaspoon Worcestershire sauce
1 teaspoon prepared cream-style
   horseradish (optional)

Preheat oven to 350 degrees. In a shallow baking pan arrange chicken. Dot with margarine. Sprinkle with cardamom, salt and pepper. Bake for 1 hour or until tender. In a medium saucepan combine apples, cider, sugar, lemon juice and rind, Worcestershire sauce and horseradish. Simmer over medium-low heat until apples are tender. Pour over chicken. Bake just until heated through. Makes 6 servings.

Approx. per serving: 236.0 calories; 5.2 gr. fat; 19.83% calories from fat.

NEW ORLEANS JAMBALAYA

Jambalaya, pronounced jum-bu-lie-ya, is a rice dish from New Orleans highly seasoned and flavored with beef, pork, chicken or ham. Try our version, and see how good it can be.

2 tablespoons corn oil margarine
½ cup onion, chopped
½ cup scallions, chopped
½ cup green bell pepper, chopped
½ cup celery, chopped
2 cloves garlic, minced
2 cups chicken broth, either
   homemade or canned
1 ½ cups fresh tomatoes,
   chopped
¼ cup fresh parsley, chopped
½ teaspoon salt (optional)
½ teaspoon fresh thyme or
   ¼ teaspoon dried thyme
⅛ teaspoon black pepper
⅛ teaspoon cayenne pepper
2 bay leaves
1 cup uncooked brown rice
8 chicken breast halves,
   skinned and boned

In a stockpot heat margarine over medium heat. Add onion, scallions, green pepper, celery and garlic. Sauté for 5 minutes. Add broth, tomatoes, parsley, salt, thyme, black pepper, cayenne pepper and bay leaves; cover. Bring to a boil over medium heat. Add rice and chicken; cover. Cook over medium-low heat for 45 minutes, stirring occasionally. Remove bay leaves. Serve hot. Makes 8 servings.

Approx. per serving: 276.0 calories; 6.8 gr. fat; 22.17% calories from fat.

LEMON SPIKED CHICKEN

Juicy, tender chicken is ready to serve in minutes with the aid of a microwave oven.

6 chicken breast halves, skinned
   and boned
2 tablespoons plus 1 teaspoon
   corn oil margarine, divided
1 ½ tablespoons all-purpose flour
1 teaspoon fresh tarragon or
   ½ teaspoon dried tarragon
½ teaspoon salt (optional)
¼ pound fresh mushrooms,
   thinly sliced
¼ cup hot water
1 teaspoon instant chicken
   bouillon
½ lemon, thinly sliced
Hot cooked rice

Cut each chicken breast half into 8 or 10 strips. In a 2-quart glass casserole place 2 tablespoons margarine. Microwave on High for 1 minute. Add chicken. Sprinkle with flour, tarragon and salt; cover. Microwave on High for 4 minutes, stirring at 1-minute intervals. In a 1-quart glass casserole place remaining 1 teaspoon margarine. Microwave on High for 1 minute. Add mushrooms; toss to mix. Microwave on High for 1½ minutes, stirring after 1 minute. Add to chicken. In a small bowl combine hot water and bouillon; stir until dissolved. Pour over chicken. Arrange lemon slices on top. Microwave on High for 5 minutes or until chicken is tender. Serve over rice. Makes 6 servings.

Approx. per serving: 200.0 calories; 7.8 gr. fat; 35.1% calories from fat.

MANDARIN ORANGE CHICKEN WITH BROCCOLI

A light-tasting preparation of chicken breasts with one of our favorites from the cabbage family— broccoli—is freshened with a garnish of mandarin oranges.

¼ cup unbleached flour
1 tablespoon paprika
½ teaspoon salt (optional)
¼ teaspoon pepper
8 chicken breast halves, skinned and boned
3 tablespoons corn oil margarine
¼ cup onion, minced
1 cup chicken broth, either homemade or canned
1 cup 1% low-fat milk
1½ pounds broccoli
1 can (8 ounces) mandarin oranges, drained

In a plastic bag combine flour, paprika, salt and pepper; shake to mix. Into seasoned flour place chicken breasts 1 at a time, shaking to coat well. In a skillet over medium heat melt margarine. Add onion. Sauté over medium-high heat until tender. Add chicken. Sauté for 5 minutes on each side. Remove chicken. Add broth. Bring to a boil over medium heat. Cook for 5 minutes, stirring frequently. Add milk. Simmer for 5 minutes, stirring frequently. Add chicken; baste with sauce. Simmer over low heat for 10 minutes, basting chicken several times. Cut broccoli into florets; peel and slice stems. In a steamer or saucepan in a small amount of water steam broccoli until tender. In the middle of each serving plate arrange chicken. Arrange broccoli around chicken. Spoon sauce over chicken and broccoli. Garnish with mandarin oranges. Makes 8 servings.

Approx. per serving: 249.0 calories; 8.3 gr. fat; 30.0% calories from fat.

ORANGE-GINGER CHICKEN WITH LEEKS

1 tablespoon corn oil margarine
1¼ pounds boneless chicken breasts, skinned and cut into 1-inch cubes
2 large leeks, cleaned, trimmed and cut into julienne strips
2 green onions, chopped
1 tomato, peeled, seeded and chopped
¼ cup dry white wine
1 tablespoon fresh gingerroot, grated
½ cup fresh orange juice
1 tablespoon all-purpose flour
½ teaspoon orange rind, grated
¼ teaspoon granulated sugar
1 cup seedless green grapes
Salt and freshly ground pepper to taste

In a large heavy skillet over medium-high heat melt margarine. Add chicken. Cook over high heat for 2 to 3 minutes or until light brown. Remove chicken. Add leeks and green onions. Stir-fry until wilted. Add tomato, wine and gingerroot; mix well to deglaze skillet. In a small bowl combine orange juice, flour, orange rind and sugar; mix well. Stir into leek mixture. Bring to a boil over medium heat, stirring constantly. Simmer for 2 to 3 minutes, stirring constantly. Add chicken, grapes, salt and pepper. Heat to serving temperature. Makes 4 servings.

Approx. per serving: 258.0 calories; 6.3 gr. fat; 21.97% calories from fat.

PEACHY CHICKEN

½ cup peach preserves
½ cup water
Juice of ½ lemon
6 chicken breasts, skinned and
boned

In a small bowl combine peach preserves, water and lemon juice; mix well. In a shallow dish arrange chicken. Pour preserve mixture over chicken. Marinate in refrigerator overnight. Preheat oven to 350 degrees. Drain chicken, reserving marinade. In a baking dish arrange chicken. Bake for 45 minutes or until chicken is tender, basting frequently with reserved marinade. Serve with rice. Makes 6 servings.

Approx. per serving: 217.0 calories; 3.1 gr. fat; 12.85% calories from fat.

TARRAGON CHICKEN BREASTS

For a festive celebration dinner try our uncomplicated chicken sauté.

1 tablespoon corn oil margarine
2 shallots, minced
½ pound fresh mushrooms, sliced
½ cup all-purpose flour
Salt and pepper to taste
2 chicken breasts, skinned,
boned and halved
½ cup dry white wine
½ cup chicken broth, either
homemade or canned
2 teaspoons fresh parsley,
chopped
1 teaspoon fresh tarragon or
½ teaspoon dried tarragon

In a 10-inch skillet over medium heat melt margarine. Add shallots. Sauté for 1 to 2 minutes. Add mushrooms. Sauté for 3 to 4 minutes. Remove vegetables; keep warm. In a small dish combine flour, salt and pepper. Coat chicken with flour mixture. In the skillet sauté chicken until brown on both sides. Remove chicken; keep warm. To the skillet add wine and chicken broth, stirring to deglaze. Add parsley and tarragon. Cook over high heat until mixture is reduced to sauce consistency. Add sautéed vegetables; mix well. On a serving plate arrange chicken. Spoon sauce over chicken. Makes 4 servings.

Approx. per serving: 264.0 calories; 6.5 gr. fat; 22.15% calories from fat.

TURKEY BREAST WITH LEMON AND CAULIFLOWER

Turkey is suddenly astounding us with its versatility. A prime factor is its flavor compatibility with other foods. Try this with leftover Thanksgiving turkey.

1 cup uncooked brown rice
2 cups chicken or turkey broth,
either homemade or canned
1½ pounds boneless turkey
breast, skinned and cut into
bite-sized pieces
1 large head cauliflower,
broken into florets
2 tablespoons corn oil margarine
¼ cup unbleached flour
2 cups 1% low-fat milk
¼ cup fresh lemon juice
1 teaspoon fresh thyme or
½ teaspoon dried thyme
½ teaspoon salt (optional)
½ teaspoon pepper
1 cup fresh parsley, chopped
Paprika

Cook rice according to package directions. Keep warm. In a medium saucepan over medium heat bring broth to a boil. Add turkey to broth. Simmer for 5 minutes or until heated through; drain. Heat 2 baking dishes in a warm oven. Place turkey in 1 dish; keep warm. In a saucepan steam cauliflower in a small amount of water for 5 to 10 minutes or until tender. Place in second heated baking dish; keep warm. In a medium saucepan over medium heat melt margarine. Blend in flour. Cook until golden brown, stirring constantly. Stir in milk gradually. Cook over medium heat until thickened, stirring constantly. Whisk in lemon juice, thyme, salt and pepper. Add turkey. On a serving platter spoon rice into center. Arrange cauliflower around rice. Spoon turkey mixture over rice; drizzle a small amount of sauce over cauliflower. Sprinkle with parsley and paprika. Into a small serving dish pour remaining sauce. Serve with turkey. Makes 6 servings.

Approx. per serving: 411.0 calories; 6.9 gr. fat; 15.10% calories from fat; high fiber.

TURKEY POLYNESIAN

Try turkey in recipes calling for chicken, veal or pork. You'll be surprised how good they will taste. You will also save money and calories.

1 tablespoon cornstarch
2 teaspoons water
1 teaspoon lite soy sauce
1 teaspoon salt (optional)
1 to 1 ½ pounds uncooked turkey breast, skinned, boned and cubed
1 cup onion, sliced
1 ½ tablespoons corn oil or safflower oil, divided
1 cup celery, diagonally sliced
1 can (8 ounces) water chestnuts, drained and sliced
1 cup juice-pack pineapple chunks or tidbits
¼ cup pineapple juice
Hot cooked rice

In a small bowl combine cornstarch, water, soy sauce and salt; mix well. Coat turkey cubes with cornstarch mixture. In a skillet over medium-high heat sauté onion in ½ tablespoon oil. Add celery and water chestnuts. Cook for 2 minutes. Remove vegetables from skillet. To skillet add remaining 1 tablespoon oil and turkey. Sauté until brown. Add sautéed vegetables, pineapple and juice. Simmer for 10 minutes. Serve with hot rice. Makes 6 servings.

Approx. per serving: 188.0 calories; 4.1 gr. fat; 19.62% calories from fat.

CURRIED TURKEY AND BROCCOLI

1 tablespoon corn oil or
  safflower oil
1 tablespoon corn oil margarine
1 ½ pounds uncooked turkey
  breast, cut into ⅜-inch slices
2 medium onions, finely chopped
2 tablespoons unbleached flour
1 tablespoon curry powder
½ teaspoon salt (optional)
¼ teaspoon pepper
1 ½ cups turkey or chicken broth,
  either homemade or canned
1 cup 1% low-fat milk
5 tablespoons nonfat dry milk
  powder
3 small bunches (about 2 pounds)
  broccoli, divided into florets

In a large skillet heat oil and margarine over medium heat. Add enough turkey to make a single layer. Sauté for 1 minute on each side. Remove turkey. Repeat with remaining turkey. Keep turkey warm. In the skillet sauté onions in the pan drippings for 5 minutes. Add flour, curry powder, salt and pepper; mix well. Cook until golden brown, stirring constantly. Stir in broth. Bring to a boil over medium heat; reduce heat. Simmer for 5 minutes, stirring frequently. In a small saucepan combine milk and milk powder. Add to curry sauce. Bring to a boil. Reduce heat. Simmer for 5 minutes or until the sauce is smooth, stirring frequently. In a steamer or saucepan steam broccoli in a small amount of water until tender-crisp; drain. To the curry sauce add turkey, spooning sauce over turkey. Cook until heated through. In the center of a serving plate arrange turkey. Arrange broccoli around turkey. Spoon sauce over turkey and broccoli. Makes 8 servings.

Approx. per serving: 217.0 calories; 4.6 gr. fat; 19.07% calories from fat.

GLAZED CORNISH HENS

This recipe has the zing of mustard and the sweetness of corn syrup to make it a terrific dish hot or cold. Serve it with wild rice and a green vegetable like asparagus.

2 Cornish game hens, cut in half
  and skinned
⅓ cup light corn syrup
¼ cup prepared mustard
2 teaspoons curry powder
1 clove garlic, minced

Preheat oven to 350 degrees. Wash Cornish hens; pat dry. On a rack in a roasting pan place Cornish hens. In a small bowl combine corn syrup, mustard, curry powder and garlic; mix well. Brush Cornish hens with corn syrup mixture. Bake for 1 ½ hours, basting occasionally. Makes 2 to 4 servings.

Approx. per serving: 461.0 calories; 9.1 gr. fat; 17.76% calories from fat.

NEW ORLEANS CATFISH

Catfish, always a Southern delicacy, has recently become popular in gourmet havens across the country. Its delicate, lean white flesh makes it suitable for all methods of cooking. Catfish should be skinned before cooking.

1 pound farm-raised catfish
   fillets, cut into serving portions
Dash of pepper
2 cups cooked brown rice
2 tablespoons onion, grated
½ teaspoon curry powder
6 thin lemon slices
4 teaspoons corn oil margarine
Parsley, chopped
Tabasco sauce to taste

Preheat oven to 350 degrees. Grease a 9x13-inch baking dish well. In prepared baking dish arrange fillets. Sprinkle with pepper. In a bowl combine rice, onion and curry powder; mix well. Spoon over fillets. Top with lemon slices; dot with margarine. Cover. Bake for 25 to 35 minutes or until fish flakes easily, removing cover for last few minutes to permit slight browning. Sprinkle with parsley. Serve with Tabasco sauce. Makes 4 servings.

Approx. per serving: 255.0 calories; 5.4 gr. fat; 19.05% calories from fat.

FISH DIJON

1 pound boneless fish fillets
2 teaspoons Dijon mustard
½ cup cooked brown rice
⅓ cup fresh parsley, chopped
⅓ cup red onion, chopped
⅓ cup green bell pepper, chopped
⅓ cup fish or chicken broth,
   either homemade or canned
½ cup part-skim mozzarella
   cheese, shredded
⅓ cup bread crumbs
Paprika to taste

Preheat oven to 350 degrees. Spray an 8x8-inch baking dish with vegetable cooking spray. In prepared dish arrange half the fillets in a single layer. Spread with mustard. Layer rice, parsley, onion and green pepper over fillets. Arrange remaining fillets over layers. Pour broth over top. Sprinkle with cheese, bread crumbs and paprika. Bake for 15 minutes. Serve immediately. Makes 4 servings.

Approx. per serving: 213.0 calories; 4.1 gr. fat; 17.32% calories from fat.

FISH FILLETS FLORENTINE

In this charming dish fish fillets transform the cheese-sauced spinach into something wonderful. Red snapper fillets are especially good in this combination. Begin the meal with a pasta dish or soup, and serve the main course ungarnished.

1½ tablespoons corn oil
 margarine
1½ tablespoons all-purpose flour
½ teaspoon salt (optional)
⅛ teaspoon pepper
1 cup 1% low-fat milk
½ cup low-fat Cheddar cheese
2 packages (10 ounces each)
 frozen chopped spinach,
 cooked and drained
2 pounds fish fillets

Preheat oven to 375 degrees. In a saucepan over medium heat melt margarine. Add flour, salt and pepper; blend well. Stir in milk gradually. Cook until thickened, stirring constantly. Add cheese. Cook over very low heat until cheese is melted, stirring constantly. In a 9x13-inch baking dish spread a layer of spinach. Cover with cheese sauce. Arrange fillets in prepared dish. Bake for 15 to 20 minutes or until fish flakes easily. Makes 6 servings.

Approx. per serving: 254.0 calories; 8.0 gr. fat; 28.34% calories form fat; high vitamin A.

MICROWAVE FILLETS PROVENÇAL

1 pound fish fillets
1 can tomatoes, drained and
 coarsely chopped
Salt and pepper to taste
¼ cup fresh parsley, chopped
¼ cup fine fresh bread crumbs
2 tablespoons green onion with
 top, minced
1 tablespoon corn oil margarine
2 cloves garlic, minced

Into a microwave-safe dish just large enough to hold fillets in a single layer spoon half the tomatoes. Arrange fillets in prepared dish. Sprinkle with salt and pepper. Cover with remaining tomatoes. In a small bowl combine parsley, crumbs, green onion, margarine and garlic; mix well. Sprinkle over tomatoes. Cover loosely. Microwave on High for 9 to 12 minutes or until fish is opaque. Let stand for 3 minutes before serving. Makes 4 servings.

Approx. per serving: 183.0 calories; 4.5 gr. fat; 22.13% calories from fat.

FISH TERIYAKI

Seafood is naturally tender and cooks very quickly. It is one of the foods the microwave oven cooks best.

2 pounds flounder fillets
¼ cup Chablis or other dry white wine
2 tablespoons teriyaki sauce
½ cup green onions, thinly sliced
2 teaspoons fresh basil or 1 teaspoon dried basil

In a shallow 2-quart glass baking dish arrange fillets. In a small bowl mix wine and teriyaki sauce. Pour over fillets. Sprinkle with green onions and basil. Cover loosely with plastic wrap. Microwave on High for 8 to 9 minutes or until fish flakes easily, turning dish ½ turn after 4 minutes. Makes 6 servings.

Approx. per serving: 153.0 calories; 1.37 gr. fat; 8.05% calories from fat.

FLOUNDER CREOLE

Creole cooking which began in New Orleans is a mixture of French, Spanish, Italian, American Indian, African and other ethnic groups. Try our taste of Louisiana with this appetizing fish creole-style.

1 cup uncooked brown rice
1 pound flounder or sole fillets
1 cup onion, chopped
1 cup green bell pepper, chopped
1 cup tomatoes, chopped
¼ cup white wine
1 teaspoon fresh basil or ½ teaspoon dried basil
½ teaspoon salt (optional)
¼ teaspoon pepper

Cook brown rice according to package directions, starting 15 minutes before preparing flounder. In a large pan with a cover place fillets. Around fillets place onion, green pepper and tomatoes. Pour wine over fillets; sprinkle with basil, salt and pepper. Cover. Cook over medium-low heat for 10 minutes or until fish flakes easily. On a serving platter arrange fillets; spoon rice around fillets. Spoon vegetables and sauce over fillets and rice. Makes 4 servings.

Approx. per serving: 315.0 calories; 2.2 gr. fat; 6.28 calories from fat.

BAKED SALMON WITH CARROT-ZUCCHINI STUFFING

The ravishing colors and subtle flavors of this dish combine to make an outstanding presentation.

1 tablespoon corn oil margarine
1 small onion, finely chopped
3 cups zucchini, shredded
1 cup carrot, shredded
¼ cup parsley, minced
1 to 2 tablespoons fresh basil or tarragon, minced or ½ to 1 teaspoon dried basil or tarragon
4 salmon steaks (4 ounces each)
1 teaspoon fresh lime juice
Salt and pepper to taste

Preheat oven to 350 degrees. In a skillet over medium heat melt margarine. Add onion. Sauté until tender. Add zucchini, carrot, parsley and basil; mix lightly. Lightly grease a 10x10-inch baking dish. Place vegetable mixture in prepared dish. Coat salmon steaks with lime juice. Arrange over vegetable mixture; sprinkle with salt and pepper. Cover. Bake for 30 minutes. Uncover. Bake for 10 minutes longer or until fish flakes easily. Makes 4 servings.

Approx. per serving: 241.0 calories; 8.7 gr. fat; 32.48% calories from fat; high vitamin A.

SALMON-STUFFED POTATOES

Simple baked potatoes lay the foundation for a savory and elegant luncheon main course or a late-night snack that is special and nutritious at the same time.

6 large potatoes, baked
2 tablespoons corn oil margarine
1½ cups fresh mushrooms, chopped
1 tablespoon fresh parsley, chopped
1 can (16 ounces) red salmon, drained
⅔ cup 1% low-fat milk
1 medium onion, chopped
Salt and pepper to taste

Preheat oven to 350 degrees. Slice tops of potatoes; scoop out pulp, reserving shells. Into a mixer bowl place potato pulp. In a skillet over medium heat melt margarine. Add mushrooms. Sauté until moisture evaporates. Add parsley. Into potato shells spoon mushroom mixture. To potato pulp add salmon and milk. Beat until smooth. Add onion and salt and pepper. Spoon into potato shells. On a baking sheet place stuffed potatoes. Bake until heated through. Garnish with fluted mushrooms. Makes 6 servings.

Approx. per serving: 284.0 calories; 8.8 gr. fat; 27.88% calories from fat.

POACHED SNAPPER

A fish is poached by cooking it briefly in simmering liquid. Firm-fleshed fish such as snapper, salmon, trout or sole—whole fish or fillets—are the best candidates for poaching. The surface of the water should be just shivering. Never boil the water.

1¼ cups Chablis or other dry
   white wine
½ to 1 cup water
1 lemon, sliced
6 sprigs fresh parsley
½ teaspoon salt (optional)
4 peppercorns
2 bay leaves
1 (1½-pound) red snapper,
   dressed and with head intact

In a fish poacher or large skillet combine Chablis, water, lemon slices, parsley, salt, peppercorns and bay leaves. Bring to a boil over medium-high heat. Add snapper. Cover; reduce heat. Simmer for 20 minutes or until fish flakes easily. To a serving plate remove snapper carefully. Garnish with additional lemon slices. Makes 3 servings.

Approx. per serving: 158.0 calories; 1.5 gr. fat; 8.54% calories from fat.

RED SNAPPER EN PAPILLOTE

Cooking "en papillote" means enclosing the food in a tight wrapping of paper or foil and baking in a hot oven until the package puffs up like a balloon. The toasty brown packages are presented on individual plates and then cut open to release the extraordinarily aromatic steam. Cooked this way, the very lean fish is fat-free. As a bonus, cooking "en papillotte" is simple. The fish can be prepared hours ahead of time,
stored in the refrigerator, brought back to room temperature and then popped into the oven before serving.

2 tablespoons corn oil margarine,
   melted
3 tomatoes, peeled, seeded
   and cut into ½-inch cubes
8 large fresh mushrooms, sliced
8 red snapper fillets
   (8 ounces each), skin removed
¾ teaspoon salt (optional)
½ teaspoon pepper, freshly ground
2 leeks, white and tender green
   part only, cut into 2-inch
   julienne strips
¾ cup fresh parsley leaves,
   loosely packed

Preheat oven to 450 degrees. Cut baking parchment or heavy duty aluminum foil into eight 18-inch squares. Fold each square in half; cut out heart shape with fold down center. Brush each heart on 1 side of fold lightly with margarine. On each margarine-brushed area place some of the tomatoes and mushrooms. Top with 1 fillet. Season lightly with salt and pepper. Add some of the leeks and parsley. Fold heart half over to enclose filling, joining edges. Fold edge over once; fold over again with a series of pleats to seal packet tightly. On a baking sheet place packets. Bake for 8 minutes. Packets will puff. To a plate remove each packet with a large spatula. Cut large cross in top of each packet with scissors or sharp knife; fold open to expose fillet. Serve with a boiled new potato and a broiled tomato half. May substitute yellowtail, grouper, flounder or pompano for red snapper. If fillets are over ½ inch thick, increase baking time. Makes 8 servings.

Approx. per serving: 268.0 calories; 5.1 gr. fat; 17.12% calories from fat.

FILLET OF SOLE WITH DILL SAUCE

4 sole fillets (4 ounces each)
1 small zucchini
1 medium carrot
2 green onions
½ teaspoon salt (optional)
1 cup (about) water
2 teaspoons cornstarch
¼ cup low-fat plain yogurt
½ teaspoon fresh dill or
¼ teaspoon dried dillweed

Preheat oven to 400 degrees. In a shallow baking dish arrange sole. Bake for 10 minutes or until fish flakes easily. Cut vegetables into strips. Spray a large skillet with vegetable cooking spray. Add vegetables and salt. Stir-fry over medium-high heat for 2 minutes. Add water; cover. Simmer for 5 minutes. Remove vegetables with slotted spoon. In a small bowl dissolve cornstarch in 1 tablespoon cold water. Stir into skillet juices. Cook until thickened, stirring constantly. In a small bowl blend yogurt and dill. Onto a serving platter layer half the yogurt mixture, sole and vegetables. Into fish pan juices blend remaining yogurt mixture. Into a sauce boat pour mixture. Makes 4 servings.

Approx. per serving: 107.0 calories; 1.5 gr. fat; 12.0% calories from fat.

Photograph for this recipe on Cover.

SOLE CALIFORNIA

2 tablespoons corn oil margarine, divided
1 pound sole fillets
2 fresh nectarines, pitted and thinly sliced
2 tablespoons fresh lemon juice
2 tablespoons fresh parsley

In a large skillet over medium heat melt 1 tablespoon margarine. Cook fillets for 2 to 3 minutes on each side or until brown. To a warm platter remove fillets; keep warm. To the skillet add remaining 1 tablespoon margarine. Add nectarines and lemon juice. Heat to serving temperature. Spoon over fillets. Sprinkle with parsley. Makes 2 to 3 servings.

Approx. per serving: 256.0 calories; 9.4 gr. fat; 33.04% calories from fat.

SOLE WITH FRESH TOMATO SAUCE

1 teaspoon corn oil margarine
3 tablespoons shallots, minced
3 tomatoes, peeled and chopped or 2 cups canned tomatoes
4 fresh basil leaves
Salt and pepper to taste
6 sole fillets (4 ounces each)

In a heavy saucepan heat margarine over medium heat. Add shallots. Cook for 2 minutes. Add tomatoes. Bring to a boil. Add basil and salt and pepper. Simmer for 10 minutes or until thickened. Preheat oven to 500 degrees. Into a blender container pour sauce. Process until smooth; strain. Keep sauce warm. Lightly brush a baking sheet with oil. On the prepared baking sheet arrange fillets in a single layer. Sprinkle with salt and pepper. With wet palms moisten tops of fillets. On the lowest oven rack place the baking sheet. Bake for 2 to 3 minutes or just until fish no longer appears raw. In a warm oven heat a serving plate. Onto the hot serving plate spoon the sauce. Arrange fillets in sauce. Makes 6 servings.

Approx. per serving: 140.0 calories; 1.8 gr. fat; 11.0% calories from fat.

SOLE POACHED
WITH TOMATOES

1 tablespoon corn oil margarine
1½ cups fresh mushrooms,
   thickly sliced
1 clove garlic, minced
3 tomatoes, seeded and
   cut into chunks
1 teaspoon fresh basil or
   ½ teaspoon dried basil
2 pinches of fresh thyme or
   1 pinch of dried thyme
1 pound sole fillets
1 can (14 ounces) artichoke
   hearts, drained and halved
Salt and pepper to taste
Granulated sugar (optional)

In a heavy saucepan over medium-high heat melt margarine. Add mushrooms and garlic. Sauté until mushrooms are tender. Add tomatoes, basil and thyme. Bring to a simmer. Add sole and artichokes; cover. Simmer for 3 minutes. Uncover. Cook for 5 minutes or until fish flakes easily. Add salt, pepper and sugar. Makes 4 servings.

Approx. per serving: 197.0 calories; 4.4 gr. fat; 20.1% calories from fat; high fiber.

SWORDFISH STEAKS IN
LIME-SOY MARINADE

6 swordfish steaks
   (5⅓ ounces each)
2 tablespoons fresh lime juice
2 tablespoons scallion, minced
1½ tablespoons lite soy sauce
1 tablespoon corn oil or
   safflower oil
1½ teaspoons Dijon mustard
1 teaspoon lime rind, grated
1 clove garlic, peeled and minced
¼ teaspoon pepper, freshly ground
1 scallion, cut into julienne strips
Lime rind, cut into julienne strips

In a glass dish place swordfish steaks. In a small bowl combine next 8 ingredients; mix well. Pour over swordfish; cover. Marinate in refrigerator for 2 to 4 hours. Preheat broiler or grill. On a broiler pan or grill place swordfish. Cook for 4 to 5 minutes on each side or until fish flakes easily. Serve with pan juices or heated marinade. Garnish with scallion and lime rind strips. Makes 6 servings.

Approx. per serving: 273.0 calories; 10.85 gr. fat; 35.8% calories from fat.

SHRIMP
CACCIATORE

2 pounds fresh shrimp, peeled
   and deveined
1 tablespoon olive oil
½ cup onion, minced
½ cup green bell pepper, minced
2 cloves garlic, minced
1 can (20 ounces) tomatoes
1 can (8 ounces) tomato sauce
½ cup red wine
½ teaspoon salt (optional)
½ teaspoon allspice
½ teaspoon fresh thyme or
   ¼ teaspoon dried thyme
¼ teaspoon black pepper
1 bay leaf, crumbled
Dash of cayenne pepper

In a large saucepan combine shrimp and boiling water to cover. Simmer for 3 minutes or until shrimp turn pink; drain. In a skillet heat olive oil over medium heat. Add onion, green pepper and garlic. Sauté until onion is tender. Add tomatoes, tomato sauce, wine, salt, allspice, thyme, black pepper, bay leaf and cayenne pepper; mix well. Simmer for 20 minutes. Add shrimp. Heat to serving temperature. Makes 6 servings.

Approx. per serving: 250.0 calories; 4.4 gr. fat; 15.84% calories from fat.

SHRIMP DIJON

Try the shrimp tossed with spaghetti for a variation.

2 pounds unpeeled fresh
   medium shrimp
2 tablespoons corn oil margarine
½ cup dry white wine
2 tablespoons fresh parsley,
   minced
2 tablespoons fresh lemon juice
1 teaspoon garlic, minced
½ teaspoon Dijon mustard
¼ teaspoon salt (optional)
Hot cooked brown rice
Parmesan cheese, freshly grated

Peel and devein shrimp; pat dry with paper towels. In a heavy skillet over low heat melt margarine. Add shrimp. Sauté for 5 minutes or until pink. Warm a baking dish in a low oven. Into the warm baking dish place shrimp; keep warm. To the skillet add wine, parsley, lemon juice, garlic, mustard and salt. Cook for 3 minutes. Place shrimp in skillet. Heat just to serving temperature; do not overcook. Serve over brown rice. Garnish with Parmesan cheese. Makes 4 to 6 servings.

Approx. per serving: 227.0 calories; 5.6 gr. fat; 22.2% calories from fat.

SHRIMP FRIED RICE

Fried rice is one of the best known of all Chinese dishes. In China it is considered a family dish of leftovers. In America we consider it a culinary achievement!

1 tablespoon Sherry
1 tablespoon lite soy sauce
2 teaspoons cornstarch
1 teaspoon granulated sugar
½ pound small peeled shrimp
2 tablespoons corn oil or
   safflower oil, divided
4 cups cold cooked rice
½ cup green onions, chopped
1 stalk celery, finely chopped
Water chestnuts, sliced (optional)
Fresh mushrooms, sliced
   (optional)
1 teaspoon fresh gingerroot,
   grated
2 eggs,* lightly beaten
Salt and pepper to taste

In a bowl combine Sherry, soy sauce, cornstarch and sugar; mix well. Add shrimp; mix gently to coat. Marinate for 1 hour. Drain. In a skillet heat 1 tablespoon oil over high heat. Add rice, green onions, celery, water chestnuts, mushrooms and gingerroot. Stir-fry until tender-crisp. Add shrimp. Stir-fry until shrimp turn pink. Remove the shrimp mixture. Add remaining 1 tablespoon oil. Add eggs and salt and pepper. Cook until set, stirring frequently. Add the shrimp mixture; mix well. Heat to serving temperature. Makes 8 servings.

* To reduce fat and cholesterol, use an egg substitute with less than 2 grams fat per serving. Fat and calorie content may vary between brands.

Approx. per serving: 219.0 calories; 5.2 gr. fat; 21.36% calories from fat.

CHINESE SHRIMP

Stir-frying cooks food quickly, and these shrimp are tender and delicious. The vegetables and their proportions can be altered to suit personal preferences.

1 tablespoon corn oil margarine
1 small onion, chopped
4 cloves garlic, minced
1 teaspoon fresh gingerroot, grated
1 cup fresh or frozen peas
6 Chinese dried black mushrooms, soaked for 30 minutes and sliced or fresh mushrooms, sliced
½ cup chicken broth, either homemade or canned
2 tablespoons lite soy sauce
2 tablespoons water
1 tablespoon cornstarch
1 pound cooked or uncooked shrimp, peeled and deveined

In a wok heat oil over high heat. Add onion, garlic and gingerroot. Stir-fry for 1 to 2 minutes. In a small bowl combine broth, soy sauce, water and cornstarch. Add to wok with shrimp. Cook until sauce comes to a boil and thickens, stirring constantly. Cook for 1 to 2 minutes longer if shrimp are uncooked or until shrimp turn pink. Serve immediately over rice. Makes 4 to 6 servings.

Approx. per serving: 202.0 calories; 4.5 gr. fat; 20.04% calories from fat.

CREOLE SEAFOOD GUMBO

You'll be dining in New Orleans with this excellent seafood stew. Gumbo filé is an herb of ground young sassafras leaves used as a flavoring and thickener in gumbos.

1 teaspoon corn oil margarine
1 cup onion, chopped
1 clove garlic, minced
7 cups water
1 pound fresh shrimp, peeled and deveined
1 package (10 ounces) frozen okra, sliced
1 cup celery, sliced
¾ cup green bell pepper, chopped
½ cup uncooked regular rice
1 can (16 ounces) whole tomatoes, undrained and chopped
1 bottle (8 ounces) of clam juice
3 tablespoons all-purpose flour
2 teaspoons Worcestershire sauce
1 teaspoon gumbo filé or
   ½ teaspoon dried whole thyme
¾ teaspoon salt (optional)
¼ teaspoon pepper
⅛ teaspoon hot sauce
1 pound fresh crab meat
1 jar (4 ounces) pimento, diced and drained

Spray a 5-quart Dutch oven with vegetable cooking spray. Add margarine; melt over medium heat. Add onion and garlic. Sauté until tender. Add water, shrimp, okra, celery, bell pepper and rice. Bring to a boil; reduce heat. Simmer, uncovered, for 30 to 35 minutes. Stir in tomatoes. In a bowl combine clam juice, flour, Worcestershire sauce, gumbo filé, salt, pepper and hot sauce; mix well. Stir into gumbo mixture. Cook over medium heat until thickened, stirring constantly. Add crab meat and pimento. Heat to serving temperature. Makes 17 cups.

Approx. per serving: 102.0 calories; 1.35 gr. fat; 11.91% calories from fat.

LEMON BARBECUED SHRIMP

For a variation, thread two shrimp on each bamboo skewer, broil and serve as appetizers. Soak the skewers in water for ½ hour to prevent them from catching fire.

2½ pounds large fresh shrimp, peeled and deveined
½ cup fresh lemon juice
⅓ cup reduced-calorie Italian salad dressing
¼ cup water
¼ cup lite soy sauce
3 tablespoons fresh parsley, minced
3 tablespoons onion, minced
1 clove garlic, crushed
½ teaspoon pepper, freshly ground

In a large shallow dish arrange shrimp. In a jar combine lemon juice, salad dressing, water, soy sauce, parsley, onion, garlic and pepper; cover tightly. Shake jar vigorously. Pour over shrimp; cover. Marinate for 4 hours. Drain, reserving marinade. Onto skewers thread shrimp. Preheat broiler or grill. On broiler pan or grill arrange skewers. Cook 5 to 6 inches from medium heat source for 3 to 4 minutes on each side, basting frequently with reserved marinade. Makes 6 servings.

Approx. per serving: 176.0 calories; 2.8 gr. fat; 14.31% calories from fat.

LEMON-GARLIC BROILED SHRIMP

2 pounds medium shrimp, peeled
1½ tablespoons corn oil margarine
2 cloves garlic, halved
3 tablespoons fresh lemon juice
1 tablespoon Worcestershire sauce
½ teaspoon salt (optional)
3 drops of hot sauce
Coarsely ground pepper to taste
3 tablespoons fresh parsley, chopped

In a 10x15-inch baking pan arrange shrimp in a single layer. In a small saucepan over low heat melt margarine. Add garlic. Sauté for several minutes; remove and discard garlic. Add lemon juice, Worcestershire sauce, salt, hot sauce and pepper; mix well. Pour over shrimp. Preheat broiler. Broil 4 inches from heat source for 8 to 10 minutes, basting once. Sprinkle with parsley. Makes 6 servings.

Approx. per serving: 206.0 calories; 4.6 gr. fat; 20.09% calories from fat.

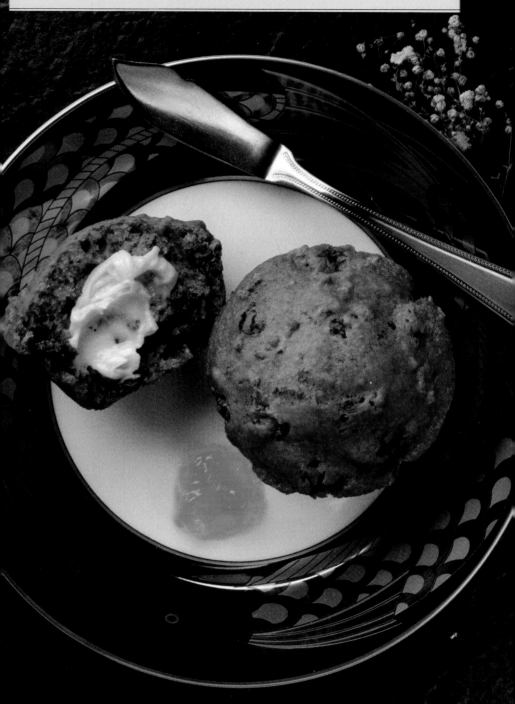

Breads

Wholesome breads constitute one of the most satisfying of all foods, and with today's electric mixers and food processors, bread making is easier than ever. Breads contain complex carbohydrates which are an excellent, steady source of energy. Also, the complex carbohydrates appear to trigger the satiety center in your brain more quickly than fat does, making you feel full more quickly. Remember, breads are not fattening—it's what you spread on them that can add calories and fat. Stay away from croissants. Croissants have a high amount of added butter and the average-size croissant has 12 grams of fat and 220 calories. To get the most nutrition from breads, bake with whole grains and unbleached flour.

Most of the recipes on the following pages will make two loaves of bread. Freeze the second loaf, wrapped in foil, until needed. To bring back that fresh-baked texture and crispness to frozen bread, simply heat foil-wrapped bread in a 350 degree oven for 20 to 40 minutes, then heat, unwrapped, for a few minutes more until the crust is crisp.

When making bread, the temperatures of liquids used in the dough are very important. Heat harms the yeast, preventing it from being an efficient rising agent. Milk or water used in these recipes should be just a little warmer than your skin temperature, no more than 115 degrees. Also, after kneading, the consistency should be soft, smooth and elastic, but not sticky. For best results, freshly baked bread should cool on a rack for at least two hours before slicing—if you, and the rest of the family, can wait that long.

Recipe for this photograph on page 141.

TRIPLE-WHEAT MUFFINS

Satisfy your sweet tooth with this nutritious home-baked snack.

1 cup whole wheat flour
1 cup all-purpose flour
1 teaspoon baking soda
1 teaspoon baking powder
½ teaspoon salt
1 egg*
1 cup buttermilk
¼ cup cracked wheat
3 tablespoons honey
2 tablespoons corn oil or safflower oil
½ cup nuts or dried dates or apricots, chopped (optional)

Preheat oven to 375 degrees. Grease 12 muffin cups or line with paper baking cups. In a large bowl combine whole wheat and all-purpose flours, baking soda, baking powder and salt; mix well. In a medium bowl beat egg lightly. Add buttermilk, cracked wheat, honey and oil; mix well. Let stand for 10 minutes. Add to flour mixture all at once; stir just until moistened. Stir in nuts or dried fruit. Spoon into prepared muffin cups. Bake for 15 to 20 minutes or until golden brown. Serve warm. Makes 12 muffins.

* To reduce fat and cholesterol, use an egg substitute with less than 2 grams fat per serving. Fat and calorie content may vary between brands.

Approx. per muffin: 150.0 calories; 3.2 gr. fat; 19.2% calories from fat.

WHOLE WHEAT MUFFINS

The batters for muffins should be mixed just until the ingredients are moistened; overbeating results in a too-dense texture. These muffins are good frozen and reheated.

½ cup all-purpose flour
2½ teaspoons baking powder
½ teaspoon salt
½ teaspoon cinnamon (optional)
1½ cups whole wheat flour
¾ cup 1% low-fat milk
⅓ cup corn oil or safflower oil
⅓ cup honey
1 egg*
1 tablespoon orange rind, grated (optional)

Preheat oven to 400 degrees. Into a medium bowl sift all-purpose flour, baking powder, salt and cinnamon. Stir in whole wheat flour. In a small bowl beat milk, oil, honey, egg and orange rind together. Add to dry ingredients; mix just until moistened. Spray muffin cups with vegetable cooking spray. Fill muffin cups ⅔ full. Bake for 15 to 20 minutes. Makes 12 to 14 muffins.

* To reduce fat and cholesterol, use an egg substitute with less than 2 grams fat per serving. Fat and calorie content may vary between brands.

Approx. per muffin: 158.0 calories; 6.5 gr. fat; 37.0% calories from fat.

Photograph for this recipe on page 139.

NATURAL BRAN MUFFINS

Bran muffins are easy to make, and everyone loves them. They are good warm or cold.

2 cups 100% bran
2 cups boiling water
5 cups unbleached flour
5 teaspoons baking soda
3 cups granulated sugar
¼ cup shortening
1 egg* or 2 egg whites
1 quart buttermilk
4 cups 40% bran flakes
1 cup mixed dried fruit with
  raisins (optional)

Preheat oven to 400 degrees. In a medium bowl combine 100% bran cereal and boiling water. Let stand until cool. In a sifter combine flour and baking soda. Into a large mixing bowl sift flour mixture. Add sugar, shortening and egg or egg whites; mix well. Add buttermilk and bran flakes; mix well. Stir in dried fruit. Grease muffin cups well. Fill the prepared muffin cups ⅔ full. Bake for 20 to 25 minutes. Makes 5 to 6 dozen muffins.

* To reduce fat and cholesterol, use an egg substitute with less than 2 grams fat per serving. Fat and calorie content may vary between brands.

Approx. per muffin: 101.0 calories; 1.2 gr. fat; 10.69% calories from fat.

WHOLE WHEAT BUTTERMILK BISCUITS

The best biscuits are those you make yourself and serve piping hot from the oven. During the baking a biscuit should rise to twice its original height. The interior should be light and tender with a crisp crust.

½ cup whole wheat flour
½ cup all-purpose flour
1 ½ teaspoons baking powder
1 teaspoon granulated sugar
¼ teaspoon baking soda
¼ teaspoon salt
3 tablespoons corn oil margarine,
  softened
7 tablespoons low-fat buttermilk

Preheat oven to 400 degrees. In a medium bowl combine flours, baking powder, sugar, baking soda and salt. Cut in margarine with a pastry blender until crumbly. Add buttermilk; mix just until moistened. Dust a board lightly with flour. Onto the floured board turn dough. Knead lightly 4 or 5 times. Roll to ½-inch thickness. Dust a 2-inch biscuit cutter with flour; cut biscuits. Spray a baking sheet with vegetable cooking spray. On the prepared baking sheet arrange biscuits. Bake for 10 minutes or until light brown. Makes 10 biscuits.

Approx. per biscuit: 80.0 calories; 3.7 gr. fat; 41.62% calories from fat.

RASPBERRY GEMS

1 ½ cups all-purpose flour
¼ cup wheat germ
¼ cup granulated sugar
1 tablespoon baking powder
1 teaspoon salt
1 cup fresh or frozen
  (without sugar) raspberries
¾ cup 1% low-fat milk
⅓ cup corn oil margarine, melted
  and cooled
1 egg,* well beaten

Preheat oven to 400 degrees. Grease 12 muffin cups or line with paper baking cups. In a bowl combine flour, wheat germ, sugar, baking powder and salt; mix well.

Add raspberries; mix well. In a small bowl combine milk, margarine and egg; mix well. Add to raspberry mixture; stir just until moistened. Fill prepared muffin cups ⅔ full. Bake for 25 minutes. Makes 12 muffins.

* To reduce fat and cholesterol, use an egg substitute with less than 2 grams fat per serving. Fat and calorie content may vary between brands.

Approx. per muffin: 141.0 calories; 5.6 gr. fat; 35.74% calories from fat.

APRICOT BREAD

This is a sweet loaf that can be enjoyed at teatime or as a snack or simple dessert.

2 cups whole wheat flour
½ cup packed light brown sugar
2 teaspoons baking soda
¼ teaspoon cinnamon
2 pounds fresh apricots, peeled and pitted or 2 cans (16 ounces each) apricots, drained
2 eggs,* slightly beaten
¼ cup corn oil or safflower oil
2 teaspoons vanilla extract
All-purpose flour

Preheat oven to 350 degrees. In a medium mixing bowl combine whole wheat flour, brown sugar, baking soda and cinnamon; mix lightly. In a blender container purée apricots. In a small bowl combine apricot purée, eggs, oil and vanilla; mix well. Add to dry ingredients, mixing just until blended; do not overmix. Spray a 5x9-inch loaf pan with vegetable cooking spray. Dust with all-purpose flour. Pour batter into the prepared pan. Bake for 55 minutes. Cool in pan for several minutes. Remove from pan. Makes 1 loaf.

* To reduce fat and cholesterol, use an egg substitute with less than 2 grams fat per serving. Fat and calorie content may vary between brands.

Approx. per serving: 191.0 calories; 6.1 gr. fat; 28.74% calories from fat.

WHOLE WHEAT BANANA BREAD

The bananas must be ripe for this dark sweet bread. This bread keeps well and can be frozen with no loss of flavor.

2 cups whole wheat flour
¼ cup wheat germ
1 teaspoon baking soda
½ teaspoon salt
1 ½ cups ripe banana, mashed
⅓ cup honey
¼ cup corn oil or safflower oil
2 eggs*
1 teaspoon vanilla extract

Preheat oven to 350 degrees. In a large bowl combine flour, wheat germ, baking soda and salt; mix well and make a well in the center. In a medium bowl combine banana, honey, oil, eggs and vanilla; mix well. Pour into well in dry ingredients; stir just until moistened. Spray a 5x9-inch loaf pan with vegetable cooking spray. Into the prepared pan spoon batter. Bake for 1 hour or until toothpick inserted in center comes out clean. Makes 1 loaf.

* To reduce fat and cholesterol, use an egg substitute with less than 2 grams fat per serving. Fat and calorie content may vary between brands.

Approx. per serving: 122.0 calories; 4.1 gr. fat; 30.24% calories from fat.

CARROT-ZUCCHINI BREAD

For best results, wrap the bread when cool, and let stand overnight before serving. This is a moist tea bread—almost like a cake.

1 ½ cups unbleached flour
½ cup whole wheat flour
⅔ cup packed light brown sugar
1 ½ teaspoons cinnamon
1 ½ teaspoons baking powder
¼ teaspoon salt
½ cup 1% low-fat milk
2 eggs *
¼ cup corn oil or safflower oil
2 teaspoons vanilla extract
1 ⅓ cups carrots, grated
⅔ cup zucchini, grated

Preheat oven to 350 degrees. In a medium bowl combine flours, brown sugar, cinnamon, baking powder and salt; mix lightly. In a blender container process milk, eggs, oil and vanilla until blended. Add carrots and zucchini. Process for 2 or 3 seconds. Add to dry ingredients; mix just until blended. Spray a 5x9-inch loaf pan with vegetable cooking spray. Pour batter into prepared pan. Bake for 45 to 55 minutes or until loaf tests done. Cool in pan for several minutes. Remove from pan. Makes 1 loaf.

* To reduce fat and cholesterol, use an egg substitute with less than 2 grams fat per serving. Fat and calorie content may vary between brands.

Approx. per serving: 179.0 calories; 5.8 gr. fat; 29.16% calories from fat.

OLD-FASHIONED MOLASSES BREAD

1 cup all-purpose flour
1 cup whole wheat flour
⅔ cup nonfat dry milk powder
½ cup packed light brown sugar
½ cup raisins
⅓ cup wheat germ
⅓ cup dried apricots, finely chopped
¼ cup nuts, chopped
2 teaspoons baking powder
½ teaspoon baking soda
½ teaspoon salt
3 eggs *
¾ cup fresh orange juice
2 bananas, cut up
½ cup corn oil or safflower oil
½ cup molasses

Preheat oven to 325 degrees. In a large bowl combine flours, dry milk powder, brown sugar, raisins, wheat germ, apricots, nuts, baking powder, baking soda and salt; mix lightly. In a food processor fitted with metal blade or in a blender container place eggs. Process until foamy. Add orange juice, bananas, oil and molasses. Process until blended. Add to dry ingredients, stirring just until moistened. Grease two 4x8-inch loaf pans. Spoon batter into the prepared pans. Bake for 1 hour or until firm. Cool in pan on wire rack. Remove from pan. Makes 2 loaves.

* To reduce fat and cholesterol, use an egg substitute with less than 2 grams fat per serving. Fat and calorie content may vary between brands.

Approx. per serving: 100.0 calories; 3.6 gr. fat; 32.4% calories from fat.

WHOLE WHEAT IRISH SODA BREAD

3 cups whole wheat flour
1 cup all-purpose flour
2 tablespoons granulated sugar
2 teaspoons baking powder
1 ½ teaspoons baking soda
1 teaspoon salt

2 tablespoons corn oil margarine
1 ¾ cups buttermilk or
  1 ¾ cups 1% low-fat milk
  plus 2 tablespoons vinegar

Preheat oven to 350 degrees. Grease a baking sheet. In a large bowl combine whole wheat and all-purpose flours, sugar, baking powder, baking soda and salt; mix well. With a pastry blender, cut in margarine until crumbly. Add buttermilk; mix well. Dough will be soft. Dust a board lightly with flour; onto the floured surface turn dough. Knead 10 times or until smooth; shape into ball. Onto the prepared baking sheet place dough ball; flatten to 2½-inch thickness. Cut a large cross about ¼ inch deep in top. Bake for 1 hour or until toothpick inserted in center comes out clean. Makes 1 loaf.

Approx. per serving: 133.0 calories; 2.1 gr. fat; 14.21% calories from fat.

NEW YORK CITY BAGELS

Sometimes called "an unsweetened doughnut with rigor mortis," bagels began as a characteristic part of the Jewish culture, especially in New York City. They are now found everywhere in the United States. They are an unusual bread because they are simmered in water before baking.

1 cup warm 1% low-fat milk,
  105 to 115 degrees, divided
1 package dry yeast
2½ tablespoons granulated
  sugar, divided
2 eggs*
2 tablespoons corn oil or
  safflower oil
1 teaspoon salt
3½ to 4 cups bread flour
1 egg white
Poppy seed (optional)

Sesame seed (optional)
Onion, chopped and sautéed,
  (optional)

In a medium mixing bowl combine ½ cup warm milk, yeast and 1 tablespoon sugar; mix well. Let stand for 5 minutes. Add eggs, oil and salt; beat well. Add bread flour and enough remaining ½ cup warm milk to make a stiff dough. Dust a board with flour. Onto floured board turn dough. Knead until smooth and elastic. Grease a bowl. Into the prepared bowl place dough, turning to grease surface; cover with plastic wrap. Let rise for 40 minutes or until doubled in bulk. Divide into 18 portions; cover with a towel. Shape each portion into ring; flatten into 2½-inch circle. With well-floured index finger make or enlarge a hole in the center of each, plumping bagels as the hole is stretched. Let rest for 20 minutes. In a large saucepan combine 3 quarts water and the remaining 1½ tablespoons sugar. Bring to a boil over high heat. Into the simmering water drop bagels 3 at a time. Poach for 3 to 4 minutes; turn bagels. Cook for 3 minutes longer, enlarging holes with handle of wooden spoon if necessary. Preheat oven to 375 degrees. Grease a baking sheet. With a slotted spoon remove the bagels to the prepared baking sheet. Brush with egg white; press poppy seed or sesame seed onto tops. Bake for 30 minutes. Spoon onion over tops after 20 minutes if desired. Makes 18 bagels.

* To reduce fat and cholesterol, use an egg substitute with less than 2 grams fat per serving. Fat and calorie content may vary between brands.

Approx. per bagel: 124.0 calories; 2.3 gr. fat; 16.69% calories from fat.

NEW WAVE PIZZA

Everyone loves pizza. Now you can make the most delicious pizza you ever tasted, and you don't have to send out for it!

1 cup warm water,
   105 to 115 degrees
1 package dry yeast
3 to 3½ cups whole wheat flour,
   divided
2 tablespoons olive oil
½ teaspoon salt
Cornmeal
½ pound part-skim mozzarella
   cheese, thinly sliced
1½ pounds fresh tomatoes,
   seeded and coarsely chopped
   or 1 cup canned tomatoes,
   drained and coarsely chopped
2 cloves garlic, minced
5 or 6 fresh basil leaves, coarsely
   shredded or 1 teaspoon dried
   basil or oregano
Salt and freshly ground pepper
   to taste
2 tablespoons Parmesan cheese,
   freshly grated (optional)
2 teaspoons olive oil (optional)

In a medium bowl combine water and yeast; stir until dissolved. Add 1 cup flour, olive oil and salt; mix well with a wooden spoon. Mix in 1 cup flour. On a working surface sprinkle 1 cup flour. On the floured surface knead dough until smooth and elastic, adding remaining ½ cup flour if necessary. Lightly flour a 2-quart bowl. In the floured bowl place dough; turn to coat surface. Cover with plastic wrap. Let rise for 1 hour or until doubled in bulk. Knead for 1 minute. Preheat oven to 500 degrees. Sprinkle a large pizza pan with cornmeal. Roll or stretch dough into a thin circle; place in prepared pan. Layer mozzarella cheese, tomatoes, garlic, basil, salt, pepper, Parmesan cheese and olive oil over dough. Bake for 10 to 15 minutes or until crust is golden. Cut into wedges. Makes 12 slices.

Approx. per slice: 193.0 calories; 7.0 gr. fat; 32.64% calories from fat; high fiber.

PITA BREAD

Light brown and puffed in the center, these Middle Eastern breads will be crusty when cool but will soften when wrapped in foil or plastic. Simply split, and fill with a favorite filling. Pitas are extremely good filled with salads or shish kebab.

2 cups warm water,
   105 to 115 degrees
1 package dry yeast
1 teaspoon salt
4½ cups unsifted all-purpose flour

In a large bowl mix water and yeast. Add salt. Add flour gradually, mixing well until smooth. Scrape side of bowl; cover lightly. Let rise in a warm place for 1 hour or until doubled in bulk. Stir dough down. Dust a board with flour. On the floured board place the dough. Divide into 12 portions; cover lightly. Let rest for 30 minutes. Dust a baking sheet with flour. On the prepared baking sheet place 2 portions. Flatten each portion lightly into 5-inch round, forcing any air bubbles to center of rounds. Preheat oven to 350 degrees. Place baking sheet on lowest oven rack. Bake for 20 minutes or until puffed but not brown. Repeat with remaining portions. Preheat broiler. Broil baked pitas for 1 minute. Makes 12 pitas.

Approx. per pita: 172.0 calories; 0.4 gr. fat; 2.09% calories from fat.

SHREDDED WHEAT ROLLS

1 cup warm water,
  105 to 115 degrees
1 package dry yeast
1 egg*
3 tablespoons granulated sugar
2 tablespoons corn oil or
  safflower oil
½ teaspoon salt
3 to 3½ cups all-purpose flour,
  divided
¾ cup shredded wheat biscuits,
  crumbled

In a large mixer bowl combine warm water and yeast; mix well. Add egg, sugar, oil, salt and 1½ cups flour. Beat at low speed of electric mixer until smooth. Add shredded wheat; mix well. Stir in enough remaining 1½ to 2 cups flour to make a very soft dough. Spray a large bowl with vegetable cooking spray. Into the prepared bowl place the dough, turning to grease surface; cover. Let rise in a warm 85-degree draft-free place for 1 hour or until doubled in bulk. Spray muffin cups with vegetable cooking spray. Dust a working surface with flour. On the floured surface knead the dough 4 or 5 times. Shape into 1-inch balls. Place 3 balls in each prepared muffin cup; cover. Let rise in a warm draft-free place for 40 minutes or until doubled in bulk. Preheat oven to 400 degrees. Bake for 12 to 15 minutes or until brown. Makes 18 rolls.

* To reduce fat and cholesterol, use an egg substitute with less than 2 grams fat per serving. Fat and calorie content may vary between brands.

Approx. per roll: 118.0 calories; 2.0 gr. fat; 15.25% calories from fat.

WHOLE WHEAT ROLLS

¼ cup corn oil or safflower oil
2 tablespoons plus 1 teaspoon
  granulated sugar, divided
½ teaspoon salt
¾ cup warm water,
  110 to 115 degrees
1 egg,* slightly beaten
1½ cups all-purpose flour
1 cup whole wheat flour
½ cup graham cracker crumbs

In a large bowl combine oil, 2 tablespoons sugar and salt; set aside. In a small bowl combine water, yeast and remaining 1 teaspoon sugar; mix well. Add yeast mixture and egg to oil mixture. Add all-purpose and whole wheat flours and graham cracker crumbs; mix well. Spray a large bowl with vegetable cooking spray. Place dough in the prepared bowl, turning to grease surface. Let rise in a warm 85-degree draft-free place for 1 hour or until doubled in bulk. Dust working surface lightly with flour. On the floured surface roll dough to ¼-inch thickness. Dust a 2¼-inch biscuit cutter with flour. With the floured cutter cut biscuits. Spray baking sheets with vegetable cooking spray. On the prepared baking sheets arrange biscuits. Let rise in a warm draft-free place for 45 minutes or until doubled in bulk. Preheat oven to 350 degrees. Bake for 15 to 20 minutes. Makes about 2 dozen rolls.

* To reduce fat and cholesterol, use an egg substitute with less than 2 grams fat per serving. Fat and calorie content may vary between brands.

Approx. per roll: 82.0 calories; 2.8 gr. fat; 30.73% calories from fat.

RUSSIAN BLACK BREAD

¼ cup warm water,
  105 to 115 degrees
1 package dry yeast
2 teaspoons granulated sugar
1 ½ cups bread flour
¾ cup rye flour
¾ cup yellow cornmeal
¼ cup instant nonfat dry milk
  powder
2 tablespoons unsweetened
  cocoa
2 tablespoons unsalted butter,
  softened
2 tablespoons fresh lemon juice
2 teaspoons instant freeze-dried
  coffee crystals
2 teaspoons caraway seed
1 ½ teaspoons salt
2 large eggs, * divided

In a small bowl combine water, yeast and sugar; mix well. Let stand until foamy. In a large mixer bowl combine bread flour, rye flour, cornmeal, dry milk powder, cocoa, butter, lemon juice, coffee crystals, caraway seed, salt and 1 egg. Add yeast mixture. With the paddle attachment beat mixture at low speed of electric mixer for 2 to 3 minutes. Replace paddle with dough hook. Knead at low speed of electric mixer for 2 minutes. Knead at medium speed for 2 minutes. Add enough additional flour if dough is sticky or water if dough is dry, 1 tablespoon at a time, to make a medium dough. Oil a large bowl. In prepared bowl place dough, turning to oil surface; cover. Let rise in a warm place for 1¾ hours or until doubled in bulk. Dust a board with flour. Onto the floured board turn the dough; punch down. Shape into a 10-inch oval. Grease a baking sheet; sprinkle with additional cornmeal. On the prepared baking sheet place the loaf; cover. Let rise for 1½ hours or until doubled in bulk.

Preheat oven to 375 degrees. Make 3 slashes on top of loaf. Brush with remaining egg. Bake for 30 minutes or until loaf sounds hollow when tapped on bottom. On a wire rack cool bread. Makes 1 loaf.

* To reduce fat and cholesterol, use an egg substitute with less than 2 grams fat per serving. Fat and calorie content may vary between brands.

Approx. per serving: 109.0 calories; 2.4 gr. fat; 19.8% calories from fat.

BREAD WREATH

This is a lovely bread to serve at holiday time.

1 ½ cups water, divided
2 ¼ teaspoons granulated sugar
1 ½ teaspoons sea salt
1 tablespoon corn oil margarine
1 package dry yeast
3 cups all-purpose flour
1 teaspoon cornstarch

In a saucepan combine 1 cup water, sugar and salt. Heat to lukewarm over low heat. Add margarine; stir until melted. Into a large bowl pour the mixture. Add yeast; stir until dissolved. Add flour; mix well. Dust a working surface with flour. Onto the floured surface turn the dough. Knead for 10 minutes or until smooth and elastic. Grease a large bowl. Into the greased bowl place the dough, turning to grease surface; cover with plastic wrap or towel. Let rise for 1½ hours or until doubled in bulk. Punch dough down. Dust a working surface with flour. Onto the floured surface turn dough. Set aside a 4½-ounce portion of dough. Divide remaining dough into 3 equal portions. Shape each into a ball;

cover. Let rest for 10 minutes. Shape each portion into ½x22-inch rope. Braid the ropes together. Grease a baking sheet and the outside of a 6-inch round baking pan. On the greased baking sheet place the 6-inch round baking pan. Shape braid around pan; moisten and seal ends together. Shape 4 ounces of the reserved dough into a ½x25-inch rope. Shape as for bow. Where the braid ends join place bow. Shape remaining ½ ounce dough into a 6-inch rope. Across center of bow and around wreath place rope; cover. Let rise for 35 minutes or until almost doubled in bulk. Preheat oven to 375 degrees. In a small saucepan mix remaining ½ cup water and cornstarch. Bring to a boil over medium-high heat, stirring constantly. Cool. Brush over wreath. (For a shinier finish use an egg wash glaze of 1 egg yolk* beaten with 1 teaspoon cream.) Bake wreath for 35 to 40 minutes or until golden brown. Makes 1 wreath.

* To reduce fat and cholesterol, use an egg substitute with less than 2 grams fat per serving. Fat and calorie content may vary between brands.

Approx. per serving: 98.5 calories; 0.36 gr. fat; 3.28% calories from fat.

CRACKED-UP WHEAT BREAD

Cracked wheat is not ground but cut. Used as a cooked cereal, it adds a crunchy texture and nutty flavor to breads.

¾ cup uncooked cracked wheat
4 to 5 cups all-purpose flour, divided
2 packages dry yeast
¼ cup packed light brown sugar
4 teaspoons salt
2½ cups warm water, 120 to 130 degrees
2 tablespoons corn oil or safflower oil
2 cups whole wheat flour

In a saucepan combine cracked wheat and water to cover. Cook according to package directions for 30 minutes; drain and set aside. In a large mixer bowl combine 2¼ cups all-purpose flour, yeast, brown sugar and salt; mix well. Add warm water and oil. Beat at low speed of electric mixer until moistened. Beat at medium speed for 3 minutes. Add whole wheat flour and cracked wheat gradually. Stir in enough remaining all-purpose flour to make a firm dough. Dust a working surface with flour. Onto the floured surface turn the dough. Knead for 5 to 8 minutes or until smooth and elastic. Grease a large bowl. Into the greased bowl place the dough, turning to grease surface; cover. Let rise in a warm place for 1 hour or until doubled in bulk. Punch dough down. Divide into 2 to 5 portions. Shape each portion into a round or oblong loaf. Sprinkle with additional uncooked cracked wheat. Grease baking sheets. On the prepared baking sheets arrange loaves; cover. Let rise for 30 minutes or until doubled in bulk. Preheat oven to 375 degrees. Bake for 25 to 30 minutes or until golden brown. On wire rack place loaves to cool. Makes 2 large or 5 small loaves.

Approx. per serving: 100.0 calories; 1.0 gr. fat; 9.0% calories from fat.

CRACKED WHEAT BREAD

This is a crunchy, rather solid bread that is moist and crumbly. It keeps well and is excellent toasted.

½ cup uncooked cracked wheat
5 to 6 cups unbleached flour or
  bread flour, divided
⅓ cup nonfat dry milk powder
3 tablespoons granulated sugar
2 packages dry yeast
4 teaspoons salt
2 cups hot tap water
3 tablespoons corn oil margarine

In a saucepan combine cracked wheat and water to cover. Cook according to package directions for 30 minutes; drain. In a mixer bowl combine 2 cups flour, dry milk powder, sugar, yeast and salt; mix well. In a bowl mix hot water and margarine. Add to flour mixture gradually, beating constantly at low speed of electric mixer. Beat at medium speed for 2 minutes. Beat in enough remaining flour to make a soft dough that pulls from side of bowl. Dust a working surface with flour. On the floured surface knead for 5 minutes or until smooth and elastic. Oil a large bowl. Place dough in the prepared bowl; turn to oil surface. Cover tightly. Let rise for 1½ hours or until doubled in bulk. Punch dough down. Divide into 2 portions; shape into loaves. Butter 2 loaf pans. Into the prepared loaf pans place loaves; cover. Let rise for 1 hour or until doubled in bulk. Preheat oven to 400 degrees. Bake loaves for 40 minutes or until loaves test done. Remove from pans. On wire racks place loaves to cool. Makes 2 loaves.

Approx. per serving: 95.0 calories; 1.26 gr. fat; 11.93% calories from fat.

FRENCH BREAD

1 ½ cups warm water, divided,
  100 to 115 degrees
1 package dry yeast
1 teaspoon granulated sugar
4 cups all-purpose flour
2 teaspoons salt
Cornmeal

In a small bowl combine ¼ cup water, yeast and sugar. Let stand for several minutes to proof. In a large bowl combine flour and salt; mix well. Add yeast mixture and remaining 1¼ cups water; mix well. Dough will be soft and slightly sticky. Dust a board lightly with flour. Onto the floured board turn dough. Let rest for several minutes. With a pastry scraper begin kneading dough, adding flour as necessary. Knead with hands for 10 minutes or until smooth and elastic. Coat a large bowl with oil. Into the prepared bowl place dough, turning to oil surface; cover with plastic wrap and a towel. Let rise in a warm draft-free place for 3 hours or until increased 2½ times in bulk. Punch dough down. Let rise for 1½ hours or until doubled in bulk. Dust a board lightly with flour. Onto the floured board turn the dough. Knead for several minutes. Cut into 2 or 4 equal portions. Cover. Let rest for several minutes. Dust a pastry cloth or board with flour. On the prepared cloth flatten 1 portion of the dough. Make a trench down center of dough; fold over and pinch edges together. Repeat process 2 more times. Shape into loaf. Repeat with remaining dough portions. Let stand on pastry cloth for 1 hour or until loaves appear swollen. Preheat oven to 400 degrees. Sprinkle baking sheets with cornmeal. Onto prepared baking sheets roll loaves. With a sharp knife or razor slash loaves. On the bottom oven rack place a pan of hot water. Bake bread for 30 to 40 minutes or until brown and loaves sound hollow when tapped.

Makes 2 large loaves or 4 baguettes.

Approx. per serving: 109.0 calories; 0.87 gr. fat; 7.0% calories from fat.

HERBED FRENCH BREAD

This bread may be made by hand or in an electric mixer equipped with a dough hook. If you have a peel and a baking stone, allow bread to rise on a peel dusted with cornmeal and slide onto the preheated baking stone. The loaves may also be baked in French bread pans.

6 cups unbleached or bread flour, divided
¼ cup fresh parsley, finely chopped
2 packages dry rapid rise yeast
2 tablespoons fresh basil, chopped or 1 tablespoon dried basil
2 tablespoons fresh chives, finely chopped or 1 tablespoon dried chives
2 teaspoons fresh rosemary, finely chopped or 1 teaspoon dried rosemary
2 teaspoons salt
2¼ cups hot water, 120 to 130 degrees

In a food processor container fitted with plastic dough blade place 5 cups flour. Add parsley, yeast, basil, chives, rosemary and salt. Begin processing. Add water gradually, processing constantly. Add enough remaining 1 cup flour to make a non-sticky dough that loosens from sides of container.

Dust a board lightly with flour. Onto the floured board turn the dough. Knead until smooth and elastic. Dust a large bowl lightly with flour. Place dough in the prepared bowl; cover. Let rise in a warm draft-free place for 30 to 40 minutes or until doubled in bulk. Punch dough down; knead briefly. Return to bowl. Let rise for 30 minutes or until doubled in bulk. Dust a board lightly with flour. Onto the floured board turn the dough. Knead several times. Divide into 2 portions. Shape each into a 15-inch long loaf. On an ungreased baking sheet place loaves side by side; cover with cloth. Let rise for 15 minutes or until risen slightly but not doubled in bulk. Preheat oven to 400 degrees. With a razor blade cut 3 diagonal parallel slashes in the top of each loaf. On bottom oven rack place baking sheet. On bottom of oven place 2 ice cubes to create steam to produce loaves with a crisp crust. Bake for 45 minutes or until golden brown.

Makes 2 loaves.

Approx. per serving: 77.0 calories; 0.2 gr. fat; 2.33% calories from fat.

SWEDISH LIMPA BREAD

This bread is popular in Scandinavia because of the distinctive flavors of fennel, orange, honey and aniseed. The finished bread has a good texture and an attractive appearance.

**2½ cups warm water,
105 to 115 degrees
2 packages dry yeast
2½ cups rye flour
3 to 4 cups bread or unbleached
flour, divided
½ cup chopped fresh orange
sections and rind
¼ cup corn oil margarine,
softened
¼ cup packed light brown sugar
3 tablespoons honey
1 tablespoon fennel seed
2 teaspoons aniseed
1 egg white
1 teaspoon water**

In a large bowl combine 2½ cups warm water and yeast; mix well. Let stand for several minutes. Add rye flour, 2½ cups bread flour, orange, margarine, brown sugar, honey, fennel seed and aniseed; beat until thoroughly blended. Add enough remaining ½ to 1½ cups bread flour to make easy to handle dough. Dust work surface lightly with flour. On the floured surface knead the dough for 10 minutes or until smooth and elastic. Grease a large bowl. Into the prepared bowl place the dough, turning to grease surface; cover. Let rise for 1½ hours or until doubled in bulk. Onto the floured surface turn the dough. Divide into 3 portions. Shape each portion into an oval. Grease a baking sheet or sprinkle a bread paddle with cornmeal. On the prepared baking sheet or paddle place the loaves. With a skewer pierce each loaf 12 times to a depth of ½ inch; cover lightly. Let rise for 40 minutes. Preheat oven to 350 degrees. Preheat a baking stone if desired. In a small bowl combine egg white and 1 teaspoon water. Brush over loaves. On the middle oven rack place the baking sheet or from the paddle onto the preheated stone transfer the loaves. Bake for 45 minutes. On a wire rack cool loaves. Makes 2 loaves.

Approx. per serving: 109.0 calories; 1.55 gr. fat; 12.79% calories from fat.

EASY LAVOSH

This Middle Eastern crisp flatbread is simple to make, keeps well and is very good in flavor and texture. It is a pleasant accompaniment to almost any type of food. It keeps best in a tightly covered container. It is very easy to make in a food processor, but it may be made in an electric mixer equipped with a dough hook or by hand.

**⅓ cup warm water,
105 to 115 degrees
1 package dry yeast
1 teaspoon granulated sugar
⅓ cup plus ¼ cup cold water,
divided
2 cups (about) bread flour
1 tablespoon butter
1 teaspoon salt
1 large egg *
2 tablespoons sesame seed,
divided**

In a small bowl combine warm water, yeast and sugar; mix well. Let stand for 5 minutes. Add ⅓ cup cold water. In a food processor fitted with bread blade combine 2 cups bread flour, butter and salt.

Process for 20 seconds. Pour yeast mixture through the feed tube. Process constantly until the mixture forms a ball, adding a small amount of additional flour if the dough is sticky. Process for 45 seconds. Grease a large bowl. Into the greased bowl place dough, turning to coat surface; cover. Let rise for 1 hour or until doubled in bulk. Punch dough down. Divide the dough into 4 portions. Shape each portion into a ball; cover. Let rest for 10 minutes. Preheat oven to 400 degrees. Dust a board with flour. On the floured board roll each portion into a 13-inch circle. On an ungreased baking sheet place each circle. In a small bowl combine egg and remaining ¼ cup cold water. Brush each circle with egg mixture. Sprinkle each with 1½ teaspoons sesame seed; prick with a fork. On bottom rack of oven place 1 baking sheet. Bake for 4 minutes. Move the baking sheet to top rack of oven. Bake for 4 minutes or until golden brown. Repeat with remaining bread. Cool. In an airtight container store bread for up to 6 to 8 weeks. Makes 4 loaves.

* To reduce fat and cholesterol, use an egg substitute with less than 2 grams fat per serving. Fat and calorie content may vary between brands.

Approx. per serving: 307.0 calories; 7.0 gr. fat; 20.52% calories from fat.

OLD-FASHIONED OATMEAL BREAD

This excellent loaf of oatmeal bread has a moist texture and a pleasing bite. Don't use instant oatmeal in this recipe.

1 cup rolled oats
1 cup boiling water
½ cup warm water,
   105 to 115 degrees
2 packages dry yeast
1 teaspoon granulated sugar
1 cup warm 1% low-fat milk
¼ cup packed dark brown sugar
1 tablespoon salt
4 to 5 cups (about) bread flour,
   divided

In a saucepan combine oats and boiling water. Cook over low heat until thickened, stirring constantly. Let stand until cool. In a small bowl combine warm water, yeast and granulated sugar; mix well. In a large bowl combine oatmeal, milk, brown sugar, salt and yeast mixture; mix well. Add 4 cups bread flour 1 cup at a time, mixing well after each addition. Add enough remaining 1 cup flour to make a medium dough. Shape into ball. Grease a large bowl well. In the prepared bowl place the dough, turning to grease surface; cover. Let rise for 1 to 1½ hours or until doubled in bulk. Punch dough down. Shape into 2 loaves. Grease two 5x9-inch loaf pans. Into the prepared pans place loaves; cover. Let rise until doubled in bulk. Preheat oven to 375 degrees. Bake for 45 to 50 minutes. Remove from pans. On a wire rack cool bread. Makes 2 loaves.

Approx. per serving: 79.0 calories; 0.4 gr. fat; 4.55% calories from fat.

OATMEAL BREAD

The addition of oatmeal to bread dough produces a tasty loaf that makes scrumptious toast.

**1 cup plus 2 tablespoons
1% low-fat milk, scalded
3 tablespoons honey
2 tablespoons corn oil margarine
1 ¼ teaspoons salt
¼ cup warm water,
   105 to 115 degrees
1 package dry yeast
1 cup uncooked regular oats
3 to 3 ¼ cups all-purpose flour,
   divided**

In a small bowl combine scalded milk, honey, margarine and salt, stirring until margarine melts. Cool to 105 to 115 degrees. In a large bowl combine water and yeast; mix well. Let stand for 5 minutes. Add milk mixture, oats and 2 cups flour; mix well. Stir in enough remaining 1 to 1 ¼ cups flour to make a soft dough. Dust work surface lightly with flour. On the floured surface knead dough for 8 to 10 minutes or until smooth and elastic. Spray a large bowl with vegetable cooking spray. Into the prepared bowl place the dough; cover. Let rise in a warm 85-degree draft-free place for 1 hour or until doubled in bulk. Punch dough down. Dust a board lightly with flour. Onto the board turn dough. Roll into a 9x15-inch rectangle. Roll as for jelly roll from narrow edge. Pinch seam and ends together. Spray a 5x9-inch loaf pan with vegetable cooking spray. Place dough in the prepared pan; cover. Let rise for 50 minutes or until doubled in bulk. Preheat oven to 375 degrees. Bake bread for 40 to 45 minutes or until loaf sounds hollow when tapped with knuckles. Remove from pan. On a wire rack cool bread. Makes 1 loaf.

Approx. per serving: 129.0 calories; 1.9 gr. fat; 13.25% calories from fat.

OATMEAL COTTAGE LOAVES

This double-decker round loaf with a hole hollowed out through the center comes from England where it was probably improvised to econo-mize baking space in a small oven. The oatmeal gives it a moist texture. Don't use instant oatmeal.

**3 cups boiling water
2 cups uncooked regular oats
¼ cup corn oil margarine
¼ cup nonfat dry milk powder
¼ cup molasses
1 tablespoon coarse salt
½ cup warm water,
   105 to 115 degrees
2 packages (1 tablespoon each)
   dry yeast
3 to 4 cups bread flour, divided
2 cups whole wheat flour
⅔ cup raisins**

In a large mixing bowl combine boiling water and oats. Stir in margarine, dry milk powder, molasses and salt. Let stand until cooled to 105 to 115 degrees. In a small bowl combine warm water and yeast; mix well. Let stand for 5 minutes. Add to oatmeal mixture; mix well. Stir in 3 cups bread flour, whole wheat flour and raisins. Dust a working surface with flour. Onto the floured surface turn the dough. Knead in enough of the remaining 1 cup bread flour to make a medium dough. Knead for 10 minutes or until smooth and elastic. Grease a large bowl. Place the dough in the prepared bowl, turning to grease surface; cover. Let rise for 1½ hours or until doubled in bulk. Divide into 2 portions. Flatten ⅔ of each portion into 7-inch round. With a knife cut 1½-inch cross in center of each round. Shape remaining ⅓ of each portion into a ball. Place 1 ball on each round on cross marks. With thumb and fingers make hole through both pieces of dough. Grease a baking sheet. Place loaves on prepared baking sheet. Let rise for 10 minutes. Place on lowest rack of cold oven. Set temperature to 450 degrees. Bake for 40 minutes. Cover top with foil to prevent overbrowning if necessary. Makes 2 loaves.

Approx. per serving: 116.0 calories; 2.0 gr. fat; 15.51% calories from fat.

PUMPERNICKEL BREAD

There is a nut-like quality in every bite of this dark rye loaf. This heavy, rather sticky dough is a bit difficult to knead, but the finished product is worth the effort.

2 packages dry yeast
1 tablespoon granulated sugar
½ cup warm water
¾ cup cornmeal
½ cup cold water
1½ cups boiling water
3 tablespoons molasses
½ ounce baking chocolate
1 tablespoon salt
2 tablespoons corn oil margarine, melted
1 tablespoon caraway seed
2 cups potatoes, mashed
4 cups rye flour
5 cups bread flour, divided
Corn oil margarine, melted

In a small bowl combine ½ cup warm water, yeast and sugar; mix well. Let proof for 5 minutes. In a medium saucepan combine cornmeal and cold water. Stir in boiling water, molasses and chocolate. Cook over medium heat for 2 minutes or until thickened, stirring constantly. Into a large bowl pour cooked mixture; stir in 2 tablespoons margarine, salt and caraway seed. Let stand until cooled to lukewarm. Add potatoes and yeast mixture. Add mixture of rye flour and 4 cups bread flour, 1 cup at a time, mixing well after each addition. Dough will be sticky. Dust a board with flour. On the floured board knead dough until smooth and elastic, adding enough remaining 1 cup bread flour to make a firm dough. Grease a large bowl. Into the greased bowl place dough, turning to grease surface. Cover with plastic wrap. Let rise until doubled in bulk. Punch dough down. Let rest for 2 to 3 minutes. Knead for 5 minutes longer. Let rest for 2 to 3 minutes. Shape into 2 loaves. Grease a baking sheet or two 5x9-inch loaf pans. Place loaves on baking sheet or in prepared pans. Let rise until doubled in bulk. Preheat oven to 425 degrees. Bake bread for 10 minutes. Reduce temperature to 350 degrees. Bake for 40 to 50 minutes or until loaves test done. Brush with the additional melted margarine. Dough may be prepared with electric mixer fitted with dough hook. Brush unbaked loaves with mixture of 1 egg white and 1 teaspoon water for a shiny crust. Makes 2 loaves.

Approx. per serving: 129.0 calories; 1.3 gr. fat; 9.06% calories from fat.

CORN-RYE BREAD

¼ cup warm water,
105 to 110 degrees
2 tablespoons honey
1 package dry yeast
½ cup warm 1% low-fat milk,
105 to 110 degrees
¼ cup hot water, 120 to 130
degrees
2 tablespoons corn oil margarine
2 teaspoons caraway seed
1 teaspoon salt
1¾ cups rye flour
1½ cups all-purpose flour
¼ cup cornmeal
1 egg white
2 tablespoons water

In a large bowl combine ¼ cup warm water, honey and yeast. Let stand for several minutes to proof. In a small bowl combine milk, ¼ cup hot water and margarine. Add to the yeast mixture. Add caraway seed and salt. In a medium bowl combine rye flour, all-purpose flour and cornmeal; mix well. Add to yeast mixture; mix well. Dust a working surface with flour. Onto the floured surface turn the dough. Knead for 10 minutes. Grease a large bowl. Into the greased bowl place dough; cover. Let rise for 1 to 2 hours or until doubled in bulk. Shape into a loaf. Grease a baking sheet. Place loaf on prepared baking sheet. Let rise for 30 minutes. Preheat oven to 375 degrees. In a small bowl beat egg white with 2 tablespoons water. Brush loaf with egg white mixture. Bake for 45 to 50 minutes. Makes 1 loaf.

Approx. per serving: 80.59 calories; 0.87 gr. fat; 9.7% calories from fat.

ENGLISH MUFFIN LOAVES

Sliced and toasted this bread is delicious—just like an English muffin but easier to make.

3½ to 4 cups all-purpose flour,
divided
2 packages dry yeast
1 tablespoon granulated sugar
2 teaspoons salt
1 teaspoon baking soda
2 cups 1% low-fat milk
½ cup water
1½ to 2 cups whole wheat flour
Cornmeal

In a large mixer bowl combine 3 cups flour, yeast, sugar, salt and baking soda. In a saucepan over medium heat combine milk and water. Heat to 120 to 130 degrees. Add to flour mixture; beat until well mixed. Stir in whole wheat flour and enough remaining all-purpose flour to make a stiff batter. Grease two 4x8-inch loaf pans; sprinkle with cornmeal. Into the prepared pans spoon batter; cover. Let rise in a warm place for 45 minutes. Preheat oven to 400 degrees. Bake loaves for 25 minutes. Remove from pans. On wire racks cool loaves. Slice and toast. Makes 2 loaves.

Approx. per serving: 74.0 calories; 0.22 gr. fat; 2.67% calories from fat.

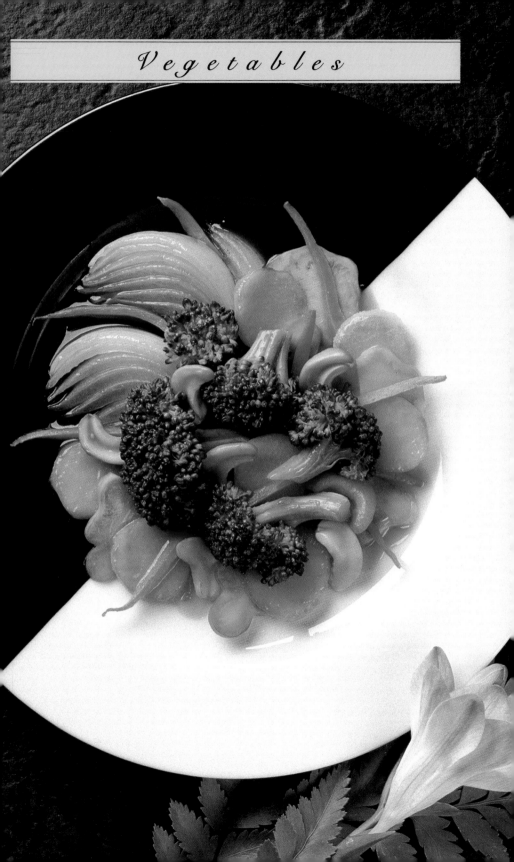

There are many methods for cooking vegetables nutritiously. As an added bonus, these cooking methods seal in flavor, color and texture.

Steaming is the best cooking method because the food cooks above—not in—boiling water, and the steam removes relatively small amounts of nutrients during the cooking process. The nutritious alternative to steaming on the range is to steam vegetables in a microwave oven.

The microwave oven is an excellent way to cook vegetables because less water and up to 70% less cooking time is needed. As a result, fewer nutrients are heat-damaged or are lost in the cooking water, unlike boiling which can decrease the vitamin A content of vegetables by 35%.

Don't overcook vegetables. They should be tender but still retain a bit of crunch. Also, don't peel vegetables, but lightly scrape them or use a vegetable brush to remove dirt. A lot of nutrients are just under the skin.

Be sure to include ample amounts of carrots, broccoli, tomatoes and Brussels sprouts in your diet because they are high in vitamin A. Vegetables and fruits provide virtually all the vitamin C (92%) and half the vitamin A (49%) in the Nation's food supply, but only 9% of the calories. The following pages provide a variety of enticing and healthy vegetable recipes.

Recipe for this photograph on page 163.

SPICED ASPARAGUS VINAIGRETTE

⅔ cup white wine vinegar
½ cup water
½ cup granulated sugar
3 sticks cinnamon
1 teaspoon whole cloves
1 teaspoon celery seed
2 pounds fresh asparagus spears,
   cooked or 2 cans (16 ounces
   each) asparagus spears, drained

In a medium saucepan combine vinegar, water, sugar, cinnamon sticks, cloves and celery seed. Bring to a boil over medium-high heat. In a shallow dish arrange asparagus. Pour hot liquid over asparagus; cover. Marinate in refrigerator overnight. Drain. Serve hot or cold. Makes 6 servings.

Approx. per serving: 113.5 calories; 1.74 gr. fat; 13.79% calories from fat.

GREEN BEANS WITH SHALLOTS

1 tablespoon corn oil margarine
2 pounds fresh green beans,
   trimmed and cut in half
2 tablespoons shallots, chopped
¼ cup water
Salt and freshly ground pepper
   to taste

In a heavy skillet over medium heat melt margarine. Add green beans and shallots. Sauté for about 2 minutes. Add water; cover. Cook for 2 minutes longer, shaking skillet occasionally. Add salt and pepper. Makes 6 servings.

Approx. per serving: 33.12 calories; 0.72 gr. fat; 19.56% calories from fat.

MUSTARD CREAM BROCCOLI AND CARROTS

2 cups chicken broth, either homemade or canned
1 pound carrots, cut into strips
1 pound fresh broccoli stems, peeled and cut into strips
3 tablespoons low-fat plain yogurt
2 tablespoons fresh watercress, finely chopped
2 tablespoons scallions, finely chopped
1 teaspoon Dijon mustard
1 teaspoon fresh lemon juice
½ teaspoon salt (optional)
½ teaspoon granulated sugar
¼ teaspoon pepper

In a medium saucepan combine broth and carrots. Simmer over medium heat for 5 minutes. With a slotted spoon remove carrots to a small dish. To the broth add broccoli stems. Simmer for 3 minutes. With the slotted spoon remove broccoli to a separate small dish. In a small bowl combine 3 tablespoons of the cooking liquid, yogurt, watercress, scallions, mustard, lemon juice, salt, sugar and pepper; mix well. Spoon half the sauce over each vegetable. Marinate each in refrigerator for several hours. On a serving plate arrange carrots and broccoli. Serve chilled or at room temperature. Makes 6 servings.

Approx. per serving: 73.0 calories; 1.0 gr. fat; 12.32% calories from fat.

BROCCOLI-CORN CASSEROLE

This easy-to-make vegetable accompaniment goes well with practically any main course. Be sure to peel the broccoli stems so they will be as tender as the florets. Cauliflower may be substituted for the broccoli for a variation.

1 bunch fresh broccoli
1 can (17 ounces) cream-style corn
½ medium onion, chopped
6 tablespoons saltine cracker crumbs, divided
1 egg,* well beaten or 2 egg whites
Dash of pepper
2 tablespoons corn oil margarine, melted

Preheat oven to 350 degrees. Separate broccoli into florets. Peel stems and cut into pieces. In a saucepan or steamer over medium heat cook broccoli with a small amount of water until tender; drain and chop. In a large bowl combine broccoli, corn, onion, ¼ cup cracker crumbs, egg and pepper; mix well. Into a 1½-quart casserole spoon the broccoli mixture. In a small bowl combine margarine and remaining 2 tablespoons cracker crumbs; toss to mix. Sprinkle over the casserole. Bake for 1 hour. Makes 6 servings.

* To reduce fat and cholesterol, use an egg substitute with less than 2 grams fat per serving. Fat and calorie content may vary between brands.

Approx. per serving: 139.0 calories; 5.6 gr. fat; 36.25% calories from fat.

BROCCOLI QUICHE

1 pound fresh broccoli
2 eggs,* beaten
¼ cup unbleached flour
2 cups low-fat cottage cheese
2 ounces part-skim mozzarella
   cheese, grated
¼ cup fresh parsley,
   finely chopped
1 tablespoon fresh lemon juice
1 teaspoon fresh basil or
   ½ teaspoon dried basil
½ teaspoon fresh oregano or
   ¼ teaspoon dried oregano
¼ teaspoon salt (optional)
¼ teaspoon pepper
⅓ cup seasoned Italian
   bread crumbs

Preheat oven to 350 degrees. Cut broccoli into florets; peel and slice stems. In a saucepan or steamer over medium heat cook broccoli with a small amount of water until tender-crisp; drain and chop coarsely. In a bowl beat eggs with wire whisk. Add flour; whisk until well blended. Add broccoli, cottage cheese, mozzarella cheese, parsley, lemon juice, basil, oregano, salt and pepper; mix well. Spray a 9x13-inch baking pan with vegetable cooking spray. Into the prepared pan pour the broccoli mixture. Top with bread crumbs. Bake for 35 to 40 minutes. Cool for 2 to 3 minutes. Cut into squares. Makes 4 servings.

* To reduce fat and cholesterol, use an egg substitute with less than 2 grams fat per serving. Fat and calorie content may vary between brands.

Approx. per serving: 277.0 calories; 8.6 gr. fat; 27.94% calories from fat; high fiber.

LEMON BROCCOLI

A perfect accompaniment to almost any entrée in the book.

2 bunches broccoli
½ cup dry bread crumbs
1 teaspoon lemon rind,
   finely grated
1 tablespoon corn oil margarine
1 clove garlic, minced
¼ cup chicken broth, either
   homemade or canned
1 tablespoon fresh lemon juice
½ teaspoon salt (optional)
⅛ teaspoon pepper

Preheat oven to 300 degrees. Separate broccoli into florets; peel and slice stalks. In a saucepan or steamer over medium heat cook broccoli florets and stems with a small amount of water until almost tender; drain. In a nonstick skillet place crumbs over very low heat. Toast until golden, stirring constantly. Into a bowl place crumbs. Add lemon rind; toss to mix and set aside. In the nonstick skillet over low heat melt margarine. Add garlic. Sauté until light golden. Add broth, lemon juice, salt and pepper. Add broccoli; toss gently to coat. Into a baking dish place broccoli; sprinkle with the crumbs. Bake for 5 to 10 minutes or until heated through; do not overcook. Makes 6 servings.

Approx. per serving: 93.0 calories; 2.9 gr. fat; 28.06% calories from fat.

MARINATED BROCCOLI

3 bunches broccoli
1 ½ cups cider vinegar
2 tablespoons fresh dill or
  1 tablespoon dried dillweed
1 tablespoon granulated sugar
1 tablespoon corn oil or
  safflower oil
1 teaspoon salt (optional)
1 teaspoon pepper
1 clove garlic, finely chopped

Slice broccoli into long pieces. Into a large bowl place broccoli. In a small bowl combine vinegar, dill, sugar, oil, salt, pepper and garlic; mix well. Pour over broccoli. Refrigerate for 24 hours. Baste broccoli with marinade; drain. Into a serving bowl place broccoli. Makes 4 to 6 servings.

Approx. per serving: 103.0 calories; 4.2 gr. fat; 36.69% calories from fat.

STIR-FRIED SESAME BROCCOLI

1 bunch broccoli
2 tablespoons sesame seed
1 tablespoon corn oil or
  safflower oil
2 teaspoons garlic, finely chopped
½ cup water chestnuts, sliced
¼ cup white wine
2 tablespoons lite soy sauce
½ teaspoon granulated sugar

Separate broccoli into florets; peel and thinly slice stems. Heat a wok over medium heat. Add sesame seed. Cook until toasted, shaking wok constantly. Remove sesame seed. Add oil and garlic. Stir-fry for 15 seconds. Add broccoli stems. Stir-fry for 4 to 5 minutes or until tender-crisp. Add broccoli florets, water chestnuts, wine, soy sauce and sugar; cover. Steam for 3 to 4 minutes or until broccoli is tender-crisp, stirring occasionally. Into a serving dish spoon broccoli; sprinkle with toasted sesame seed. Makes 4 servings.

Approx. per serving: 95.0 calories; 4.38 gr. fat; 41.49% calories from fat.

TENDER-CRISP BROCCOLI AND CARROTS

The point of stir-frying is to keep the food moving constantly so that the food comes in contact with the hottest part of the pan and cooks quickly and evenly, sealing in flavor and color. A wok is the best cooking utensil for stir-frying because the sloping sides and rounded bottom help keep the food in motion.

1 pound fresh broccoli
1 tablespoon corn oil or safflower oil
2 medium carrots, cut into matchstick strips
2 small onions, cut into wedges
1 can (8 ounces) sliced water chestnuts, drained
⅓ cup light corn syrup
3 tablespoons cider vinegar
2 tablespoons cornstarch
2 tablespoons lite soy sauce
½ teaspoon ginger
Unsalted cashews (optional)

Separate broccoli into florets. Peel and thinly slice stems. In a wok heat oil over medium-high heat. Add broccoli stems, carrots and onions. Stir-fry until tender-crisp. Add florets and water chestnuts. Stir-fry for 1 minute. In a small bowl combine corn syrup, vinegar, cornstarch, soy sauce and ginger. Stir into vegetables. Cook for 1 minute. Sprinkle with cashews. Makes 4 to 6 servings.

Approx. per serving: 226.0 calories; 6.0 gr. fat; 23.89% calories from fat.

Photograph for this recipe on page 157.

BRUSSELS SPROUTS AND CHEESE BAKE

Ten minutes from start to finish is all it takes to prepare this Brussels sprout and cheese entrée. Relax while it bakes for 45 minutes.

20 ounces fresh Brussels sprouts or frozen Brussels sprouts, thawed and drained
2 cups low-fat cottage cheese
1 cup low-fat plain yogurt
½ cup scallions, sliced
2 cloves garlic, minced
½ teaspoon paprika
½ teaspoon salt (optional)
¼ teaspoon pepper
1 cup seasoned Italian bread crumbs
2 ounces part-skim mozzarella cheese, grated

Preheat oven to 300 degrees. In a saucepan or steamer over medium heat cook Brussels sprouts with a small amount of water until almost tender; drain. In a large bowl combine Brussels sprouts, cottage cheese, yogurt, scallions, garlic, paprika, salt and pepper; mix well. Lightly oil a casserole. Into the prepared casserole spoon the Brussels sprouts mixture. Sprinkle bread crumbs and mozzarella over the top. Bake for 45 minutes. Makes 6 servings.

Approx. per serving: 221.0 calories; 4.8 gr. fat; 19.54% calories from fat.

CURRIED BRUSSELS SPROUTS

Brussels sprouts can be steamed, blanched or microwaved. Cooking time depends on the freshness of the vegetables. Test with the point of a sharp knife. They should be tender but retain a slight crunch.

1 pound fresh Brussels sprouts
1 tablespoon corn oil margarine
2 tablespoons all-purpose flour
1 tablespoon onion, minced
½ teaspoon salt (optional)
¼ to ½ teaspoon curry powder
1 cup 1% low-fat milk

Cook Brussels sprouts by your choice of method; drain and set aside. In a small saucepan over medium heat melt margarine. Add flour, onion, salt and curry powder; mix well. Stir in milk gradually. Cook until thickened, stirring constantly. Fold in Brussels sprouts. Heat to serving temperature. Makes 4 servings.

Approx. per serving: 110.0 calories; 4.1 gr. fat; 33.54% calories from fat.

HERBED BRUSSELS SPROUTS AND CARROTS

1 pound fresh Brussels sprouts
2 cups chicken broth, either homemade or canned
½ pound fresh baby carrots, scraped
1 tablespoon fresh lemon juice
2 teaspoons corn oil or safflower oil
1 teaspoon fresh tarragon or ½ teaspoon dried tarragon
Dash of nutmeg, ground

Wash Brussels sprouts; discard any wilted outer leaves. In the base of each Brussels sprout cut a cross. In a 2-quart saucepan over medium heat bring broth to a boil. Add Brussels sprouts and carrots. Bring to a boil; cover and reduce heat. Simmer for 6 to 8 minutes or until vegetables are tender; drain. Add lemon juice, oil, tarragon and nutmeg; toss lightly. Makes 6 servings.

Approx. per serving: 70.0 calories; 2.2 gr. fat; 28.28% calories from fat.

CABBAGE AND GREEN BEANS

Don't overcook the green beans— they should be bright green and still have a bit of crunch left. Overcooking also ruins cabbage, giving it a mushy texture and a strong taste.

**1 tablespoon corn oil margarine
4 cups green cabbage, shredded
½ cup vinegar
¼ cup onion, chopped
2 tablespoons granulated sugar
1 teaspoon salt (optional)
Dash of pepper
2 cups fresh green beans, cooked
  and drained or 1 package
  (10 ounces) frozen green beans,
  cooked and drained
Imitation bacon pieces
  for garnish**

In a skillet over medium heat melt margarine. Add cabbage, vinegar, onion, sugar, salt and pepper. Sauté for several minutes. Cover; reduce heat. Simmer for 15 minutes or until cabbage has cooked down to ½ the volume. Cabbage may be refrigerated until serving time if desired. Add green beans. Heat for 5 minutes or to serving temperature. Into serving dish spoon vegetable mixture. Garnish with imitation bacon pieces. Makes 6 servings.

Approx. per serving: 63.0 calories; 2.1 gr. fat; 30.0% calories from fat.

CABBAGE AND ZUCCHINI

**4 teaspoons corn oil or
  safflower oil
1 clove garlic, chopped
6 to 7 cups cabbage, sliced
2 medium zucchini, thinly sliced
1 teaspoon granulated sugar
Salt to taste**

In a skillet heat oil over high heat. Add garlic. Stir-fry for 1 minute. Add cabbage and zucchini. Stir-fry for 2 minutes. Reduce heat to medium. Add sugar and salt. Stir-fry for 7 to 8 minutes or until tender-crisp. Into a serving dish spoon the vegetables. Makes 8 servings.

Approx. per serving: 44.0 calories; 2.3 gr. fat; 47.0% calories from fat.

COLCANNON
(CABBAGE WITH POTATOES)

1 pound cabbage, chopped
2 small leeks, chopped
1 cup 1% low-fat milk
1 pound potatoes, cooked
⅛ teaspoon mace or nutmeg
Salt and pepper to taste

In a saucepan or steamer over medium heat cook cabbage with a small amount of water until tender; drain. In a saucepan combine leeks and milk. Simmer until leeks are tender. In a mixer bowl combine leeks and potatoes. Beat until well mixed. Add cabbage; beat well. Add mace, salt and pepper. Makes 6 to 8 servings.

Approx. per serving: 126.0 calories; 0.8 gr. fat; 5.71% calories from fat.

CREAMED
CABBAGE

There is nothing more satisfying than good hearty country food, and this wonderful mixture of cabbage, herbs and mustard is great with almost any main dish.

1 head (1 ½ pounds) green
   cabbage, grated
1 teaspoon corn oil margarine
1 tablespoon unbleached flour
2 teaspoons fresh thyme or
   1 teaspoon dried thyme
⅔ cup 1% low-fat milk
5 teaspoons vegetable broth,
   either homemade or canned
½ teaspoon Dijon mustard
½ teaspoon salt (optional)
¼ teaspoon pepper

In a saucepan or steamer over medium heat cook cabbage in a small amount of water just until tender; drain very well. In a large skillet over medium heat melt margarine. Add flour and thyme; blend well. Add milk and broth gradually. Cook until thickened, whisking constantly. Blend in mustard. Add cabbage; mix until coated. Cook until cabbage is tender. Season with salt and pepper. Makes 4 servings.

Approx. per serving: 73.0 calories; 1.7 gr. fat; 20.95% calories from fat.

DILLED CABBAGE

4 cups cabbage, coarsely shredded
½ cup carrots, coarsely shredded
⅓ cup chicken broth, either homemade or canned
¼ cup green onions, sliced
1 teaspoon fresh dill or
 ½ teaspoon dried dillweed
¼ teaspoon pepper
1 tablespoon corn oil margarine
½ teaspoon mustard

In a large saucepan combine cabbage, carrots, chicken broth, green onions, dill and pepper. Cover. Cook over medium heat for 5 minutes or until tender. Melt margarine in a small saucepan; blend in mustard. Drizzle over cabbage mixture.
Makes 6 servings.

Approx. per serving: 26.0 calories; 0.8 gr. fat; 27.69% calories from fat.

PURPLE PASSION CABBAGE

To retain the bright red color of red cabbage it is combined with acids such as wine, apple juice, vinegar or lemon juice. Red cabbage has a coarser texture than green cabbage and requires a longer cooking time.

2 tablespoons corn oil margarine
½ cup onion, chopped
2 pounds red cabbage, shredded
⅓ cup granulated sugar
⅓ cup cider vinegar
1 tablespoon fresh lemon juice
2 teaspoons salt (optional)
Pepper to taste

In a saucepan over medium heat melt margarine. Add onion. Sauté until onion is tender. Add cabbage, sugar, vinegar, lemon juice, salt and pepper. Cook for 20 to 30 minutes or until cabbage is tender. This dish is best made the day before serving and reheated just before serving.
Makes 6 to 8 servings.

Approx. per serving: 116.0 calories; 4.2 gr. fat; 32.58% calories from fat.

SCALLOPED CABBAGE AU GRATIN

**4 cups cabbage, coarsely
  shredded
Salt (optional)
1 can (14 ounces) tomatoes,
  undrained
2 teaspoons granulated sugar
1 teaspoon fresh oregano or
  ½ teaspoon dried oregano
Freshly ground pepper to taste
½ cup low-fat Cheddar cheese
1 cup fine bread crumbs**

Preheat oven to 350 degrees. In a saucepan of boiling water place cabbage and salt to taste. Cook over medium heat for 6 minutes or until wilted; drain. In a medium bowl combine tomatoes, sugar, 1 teaspoon salt and oregano; stir to break up tomatoes. Grease a 6-cup baking dish. In the prepared baking dish place cabbage. Sprinkle with salt and pepper to taste. Spoon tomato mixture on top. Sprinkle with cheese and crumbs. Bake for 30 minutes or until heated through.
Makes 6 servings.

Approx. per serving: 116.0 calories; 2.7 gr. fat; 20.94% calories from fat.

TWO-CABBAGE STIR-FRY

**1 tablespoon rice vinegar
1 tablespoon water
1 teaspoon lite soy sauce
1 teaspoon cornstarch
1 tablespoon corn oil or
  safflower oil
1 small onion, chopped
1 teaspoon fresh gingerroot,
  chopped
1 cup red cabbage, thinly sliced
1 cup green cabbage, thinly sliced**

In a small dish combine vinegar, water, soy sauce and cornstarch; mix well and set aside. In a wok or heavy skillet heat oil over medium heat. Add onion and gingerroot. Stir-fry for 1 minute. Add red and green cabbage. Stir-fry for 3 to 5 minutes or until tender. Add vinegar mixture. Bring to a boil, stirring constantly. Serve hot.
Makes 3 servings.

Approx. per serving: 57.0 calories; 2.7 gr. fat; 42.0% calories from fat.

GINGER CARROTS

Here's a colorful, fresh tasting side dish for roasted poultry.

½ cup granulated sugar
¼ cup fresh orange juice
¼ cup chicken broth, either homemade or canned
1 teaspoon corn oil margarine
Grated rind of 1 lemon
½ teaspoon ginger, ground
5 whole cloves
1 bunch baby carrots, trimmed and peeled

In a saucepan combine sugar, orange juice, broth, margarine, lemon rind, ginger and cloves. Simmer for 10 minutes. Add carrots. Simmer until tender-crisp. Makes 4 servings.

Approx. per serving: 157.0 calories; 1.3 gr. fat; 7.45% calories from fat.

CARROTS AND TURNIP WITH ORANGE

1 small yellow turnip (rutabaga), peeled and cut into ¾-inch pieces
4 carrots, peeled and cut into ¾-inch pieces
2 tablespoons light brown sugar
2 tablespoons frozen orange juice concentrate
1 tablespoon corn oil margarine
Pinch of nutmeg
Salt and freshly ground pepper to taste
Fresh parsley, chopped (optional)

In separate saucepans place turnip and carrots with a small amount of water. Bring to a boil over medium heat; reduce heat. Simmer until turnip and carrots are tender; drain. In separate bowls or in food processor mash each vegetable until smooth. In a medium bowl combine turnip, carrots, brown sugar, orange juice concentrate, margarine, nutmeg, salt and pepper; mix well. Sprinkle with parsley. Serve immediately. May be reheated in a covered saucepan before serving. Makes 8 servings.

Approx. per serving: 54.0 calories; 1.5 gr. fat; 25.0% calories from fat.

MARINATED CARROTS

1½ pounds carrots, sliced
2 tablespoons broth, either homemade or canned
2 teaspoons olive oil
2 cloves garlic, peeled and cut in half
1½ teaspoons granulated sugar
¼ teaspoon salt (optional)
⅛ teaspoon white pepper
½ cup fresh watercress, chopped

In a steamer or medium saucepan steam carrots with a small amount of water until tender-crisp; drain. In a medium bowl combine broth, vinegar, oil, garlic, sugar, salt and white pepper; mix well. Add watercress and carrots; mix well. Marinate in refrigerator for several hours to overnight. Serve chilled or reheat gently to serve hot. Makes 8 servings.

Approx. per serving: 50.0 calories; 1.3 gr. fat; 23.4% calories from fat.

MORE THAN CARROTS

Carrots and cabbage are an unusually good tasting combination.

¼ cup plus 3 tablespoons chicken broth, either homemade or canned, divided
3 tablespoons white wine vinegar
2 tablespoons light brown sugar
1 tablespoon cornstarch
1 teaspoon salt (optional)
1 tablespoon corn oil margarine
2 cups carrots, diagonally cut into ¼-inch slices
2 cups red cabbage, cut into ¼-inch chunks
1 cup green onions, diagonally sliced
½ teaspoon ginger, ground

In a small bowl combine ¼ cup broth, vinegar, brown sugar, cornstarch and salt; set aside. Heat a wok or large skillet over high heat. Add margarine. Add carrots, cabbage and green onions. Stir-fry for 1 minute. Add the remaining 3 tablespoons broth and ginger. Reduce heat to medium; cover. Cook for 4 minutes or until carrots are tender-crisp. Stir in the cornstarch mixture. Cook until thickened, stirring constantly. Serve hot or cold. Makes 4 servings.

Approx. per serving: 89.0 calories; 3.1 gr. fat; 31.34% calories from fat.

TARRAGON CARROTS

2 cups carrots, thinly sliced
2 small onions, thinly sliced
2 tablespoons water
1 teaspoon fresh tarragon or
½ teaspoon dried tarragon
Salt and freshly ground pepper
to taste
2 teaspoons corn oil margarine

Preheat oven to 350 degrees if not using microwave. Lightly oil a large sheet foil or a 6-cup glass baking dish. On the foil or in the dish layer carrots and onions. Sprinkle water, tarragon, salt and pepper on onions. Seal foil or cover dish. Bake foil packet for 30 minutes or microwave dish on High for 10 to 12 minutes or until carrots are tender. Stir in margarine. Makes 4 servings.

Approx. per serving: 62.0 calories; 2.2 gr. fat; 31.93% calories from fat.

CAULIFLOWER QUICHE

Biscuit mix in this recipe forms a bottom crust as the quiche cooks. For added color combine red and green peppers.

1 package (8 ounces) frozen
cauliflower
1 ¼ cups low-fat Cheddar cheese,
shredded
½ cup green bell pepper, chopped
⅓ cup onion, finely chopped
1 cup 1% low-fat milk
¾ cup egg substitute *
½ cup biscuit mix
¼ teaspoon paprika
⅛ teaspoon pepper

Preheat oven to 375 degrees. Cook cauliflower according to package directions, omitting salt. Drain and coarsely chop. Place on paper towels; squeeze to remove excess moisture. Coat a 9-inch pie plate with vegetable cooking spray. On the prepared pie plate layer cauliflower, cheese, green pepper and onion. In a blender container combine milk, Egg Beaters, biscuit mix, paprika and pepper. Process for 15 seconds. Pour over vegetables. Bake for 30 to 35 minutes or until set. Let stand for 5 minutes before serving. Makes 6 servings.

* Nutritional analysis based on using *Fleischmann's Egg Beaters* egg substitute. Fat and calorie content may vary between brands.

Approx. per serving: 218.0 calories; 9.5 gr. fat; 39.2% calories from fat.

POACHED CELERY PROVENÇAL

1 bunch celery
3 cups chicken broth, either homemade or canned
3 strips (2 inches each) orange rind
1 bay leaf
2 cups fresh tomatoes, chopped
½ cup carrots, chopped
½ teaspoon fresh thyme or ¼ teaspoon dried thyme
Pepper to taste

Wash celery well. Cut tops from celery bunch, leaving a 7-inch base. Cut base into 6 wedges. Chop ½ cup celery tops. Reserve any remaining celery tops for another purpose. In a medium skillet place celery wedges and broth; cover. Simmer over medium-low heat for 10 minutes or until tender-crisp, turning wedges once. Remove celery. Add orange rind and bay leaf. Simmer until liquid is reduced to 1¼ cups. Add the chopped celery tops, tomatoes, carrots, thyme and pepper; cover. Simmer for 5 minutes or until vegetables are tender, stirring occasionally. Add celery wedges. Heat to serving temperature. Makes 6 servings.

Approx. per serving: 36.66 calories; 0.86 gr. fat; 21.0% calories from fat.

HERBED CORN ON THE COB

Summertime means fresh corn on the cob. This recipe offers a change of pace from the usual method of preparation. It may also be cooked on the grill instead of in the oven.

4 ears fresh corn
3 tablespoons fresh dill, minced or 1 tablespoon dried dillweed
3 tablespoons fresh thyme, minced or 1 tablespoon dried thyme
1 tablespoon water
1 tablespoon corn oil or safflower oil
1 clove garlic, minced

Preheat oven to 450 degrees. Remove the husks and silk from corn just before cooking. In a small bowl combine dill, thyme, water, oil and garlic; mix well. Brush corn with mixture. On squares of aluminum foil place prepared corn ears. Wrap each ear tightly in the foil. Bake for 25 minutes, turning several times. Makes 4 servings.

Approx. per serving: 94.44 calories; 3.96 gr. fat; 38.0% calories from fat.

EGGPLANT PARMESAN

This version of the popular Italian dish is lighter and fresher than usual.

3 medium eggplant, peeled and sliced
Salt (optional)
1 tablespoon olive oil
1 ½ cups onion, finely chopped
2 cloves garlic, minced
2 cups low-fat cottage cheese
3 ounces part-skim mozzarella cheese, grated
½ cup bread crumbs
2 teaspoons fresh oregano or 1 teaspoon dried oregano
2 teaspoons fresh basil or 1 teaspoon dried basil
2 teaspoons fresh thyme or 1 teaspoon dried thyme
¼ teaspoon pepper
3 fresh tomatoes, thinly sliced
2 cups Marinara Sauce (see page 72)
2 tablespoons Parmesan cheese, freshly grated

Preheat oven to 350 degrees. Salt eggplant slices lightly. Spray baking sheet with vegetable cooking spray. On prepared baking sheet arrange eggplant slices. Bake for 15 minutes or until tender. In a skillet heat olive oil over medium heat. Add onion and garlic. Sauté until soft. Remove from heat. Add cottage cheese, mozzarella cheese, bread crumbs, oregano, basil, thyme, ½ teaspoon salt and pepper; mix well. Spray a 9x13-inch baking pan with vegetable cooking spray. In the prepared pan arrange half the eggplant slices. Spread with cottage cheese mixture; add a layer of the remaining eggplant slices. Arrange tomato slices over the eggplant. Pour the Marinara Sauce over the top; sprinkle with Parmesan cheese; cover. Bake for 25 minutes. Uncover. Bake for 10 minutes longer. Let stand for several minutes before serving. Makes 8 servings.

Approx. per serving: 215.0 calories; 7.8 gr. fat; 32.65% calories from fat.

CURRIED ONIONS AND CUCUMBER

Most people think of cucumbers as a raw vegetable but cooked cucumbers have an unusual, subtle flavor.

1 ½ cups water, divided
3 large onions, cut into eighths
1 large cucumber, peeled and chopped
¼ cup nonfat dry milk powder
3 tablespoons all-purpose flour
½ to 1 teaspoon curry powder
1 tablespoon corn oil margarine
Salt and pepper to taste

In a saucepan bring 1 cup water to a boil over high heat. Add onions and cucumber; reduce heat and cover. Simmer for 5 minutes. In a small bowl combine dry milk powder, flour and curry powder. Stir in ½ cup water gradually, blending well. Into the onion mixture stir flour mixture gradually. Cook until thickened, stirring constantly. Add margarine, salt and pepper. Makes 6 servings.

Approx. per serving: 77.0 calories; 2.2 gr. fat; 25.71% calories from fat.

SWEET AND SOUR ONIONS

A nice addition to the holiday buffet table, these onions can be prepared way ahead so you can spend the time saved basting the turkey!

1 pound small white onions
1 cup dry white wine
1 cup raisins
½ cup water
½ cup white wine vinegar
¼ cup tomato paste
2 tablespoons olive oil
2 tablespoons fresh parsley, chopped
2 bay leaves
1 teaspoon granulated sugar
1 teaspoon fresh thyme or
 ½ teaspoon dried thyme
½ teaspoon salt
Dash of pepper, freshly ground

In a large saucepan of boiling water blanch onions for 2 minutes; drain. Rinse under cold water until cool. Trim root ends; peel. In a large non-corrosive skillet combine wine, raisins, water, vinegar, tomato paste, olive oil, parsley, bay leaves, sugar, thyme, salt and pepper. Bring mixture to a boil over medium-high heat, stirring constantly. Add onions; cover. Reduce heat. Simmer for 15 minutes, stirring occasionally. Uncover. Cook for 5 to 10 minutes longer or until onions are tender and liquid is thickened. Remove onions with slotted spoon if tender before liquid is thickened, returning onions to sauce just before serving. Serve warm, at room temperature or chilled. May be stored in refrigerator for up to 1 week. Makes 6 servings.

Approx. per serving: 182.46 calories; 4.77 gr. fat; 23.52% calories from fat.

PARSNIPS IN ORANGE SAUCE

12 small parsnips, cooked
½ cup fresh orange juice
2 tablespoons light brown sugar
2 tablespoons light corn syrup
½ teaspoon salt (optional)
Pinch of paprika
1 tablespoon corn oil margarine
Freshly grated orange rind

Preheat oven to 400 degrees. In a greased shallow 8x12-inch baking dish place parsnips. In a small bowl combine orange juice, brown sugar, corn syrup, salt and paprika; mix well. Pour over parsnips. Dot with margarine; sprinkle with orange rind. Bake for 20 minutes. Makes 6 servings.

Approx. per serving: 126.0 calories; 2.0 gr. fat; 14.28% calories from fat.

BAKED POTATO CHUNKS WITH GARLIC

The flavor of garlic is strongest when mashed, crushed or forced through a garlic press. When unpeeled and cooked, garlic loses its powerful flavor and becomes mild, delicate and butter-soft.

4 baking potatoes, peeled or unpeeled
1 bulb garlic (about 10 cloves), unpeeled
2 tablespoons olive oil
Coarse salt and freshly ground pepper to taste

Preheat oven to 450 degrees. Cut potatoes into chunks. In a shallow baking pan arrange potato chunks. Add unpeeled garlic cloves. Drizzle olive oil over potatoes; spread oil to coat cut surfaces. Bake for 30 minutes or until potatoes are brown on the outside and soft inside, stirring every 10 minutes and basting with pan juices. Sprinkle with salt and pepper. Makes 4 servings.

Approx. per serving: 170.0 calories; 6.75 gr. fat; 35.7% calories from fat.

HASHED BROWNS

2 large baking potatoes
2 tablespoons onion, finely chopped
1 clove garlic, finely minced
½ teaspoon fresh thyme or ¼ teaspoon dried thyme
⅛ teaspoon pepper

In a saucepan cook potatoes in boiling water to cover until tender; drain and cool slightly. Peel and shred. In a bowl combine potatoes, onion, garlic, thyme and pepper; toss to mix. Spray a 10-inch nonstick skillet with vegetable cooking spray; place over medium heat until hot. Into the preheated skillet pack potato mixture. Cook for 6 to 7 minutes or until browned on the bottom. Onto a plate invert the potato patty. Into the skillet slip the potato patty browned side up. Cook for 6 to 7 minutes or until browned. Cut into wedges. Makes 4 servings.

Approx. per serving: 150.0 calories; 0.2 gr. fat; 1.2% calories from fat.

LIGHTLY STUFFED POTATOES

You can vary the filling with other fresh chopped herbs, such as chives, basil or thyme. Try adding a finely minced jalapeño pepper for a taste of the Southwest.

2 baking potatoes, scrubbed
1 cup low-fat cottage cheese
2 ounces part-skim mozzarella cheese, shredded
¼ cup Parmesan cheese, freshly grated
2 tablespoons fresh parsley, chopped
2 tablespoons fresh dill, chopped or 1 tablespoon dried dillweed
Freshly ground pepper to taste

Preheat oven to 350 degrees. Bake potatoes for 1 hour or until tender. Cut potatoes into halves lengthwise; scoop out pulp, leaving ¼-inch shells. Into a bowl place potato pulp. Add cottage cheese, mozzarella cheese, Parmesan cheese, parsley, dill and pepper; mix well. Spoon into potato shells. On a baking sheet place the stuffed potatoes. Bake for 15 minutes or until lightly browned. Makes 4 servings.

Approx. per serving: 146.0 calories; 5.3 gr. fat; 32.67% calories from fat.

MASHED POTATOES WITH ONIONS

A potato ricer makes the best lump-free mashed potatoes.

6 large potatoes, peeled and cut into quarters
2 teaspoons corn oil margarine
2 medium onions, finely chopped
1 tablespoon water
½ cup 1% low-fat milk, divided
Salt and pepper to taste

In a large saucepan combine potatoes and water to cover. Bring to a boil over medium heat. Cook for 20 minutes or until potatoes are tender. In a heavy skillet over medium-low heat melt margarine. Add onions and 1 tablespoon water. Cook for 10 to 15 minutes or until onions are tender but not brown, stirring occasionally. Drain potatoes. Cook over low heat for 1 to 2 minutes or until dry, shaking saucepan to prevent sticking. In a large bowl combine potatoes and ¼ cup milk. Mash potatoes. Add enough remaining ¼ cup milk to make potatoes smooth and fluffy. Into the mashed potatoes stir the onions, salt and pepper. Makes 6 servings.

Approx. per serving: 158.0 calories; 1.8 gr. fat; 10.25% calories from fat.

OVEN FRENCH FRIES

An old favorite minus the deep frying! Try a variation by using unpeeled sweet potatoes cut into sticks.

2 pounds potatoes, unpeeled, cut into large sticks
2 tablespoons corn oil or safflower oil
½ teaspoon pepper
½ teaspoon paprika

Preheat oven to 375 degrees. In a large bowl combine potatoes, oil, pepper and paprika; toss to coat well. On a nonstick baking sheet arrange potatoes in a single layer. Bake for 20 minutes. With a spatula loosen potatoes; toss potatoes gently. Bake for 20 minutes longer. With the spatula remove potatoes to a serving plate. Makes 6 servings.

Approx. per serving: 172.0 calories; 4.7 gr. fat; 24.59% calories from fat.

PARSLEY POTATOES

Small, red new potatoes and fresh parsley are combined in our eye-catching and delicious accompaniment to almost any entrée.

2 pounds small new potatoes, 1 strip peel removed around center
Salt to taste
2 tablespoons corn oil margarine
1 tablespoon fresh parsley, finely chopped

In a large saucepan combine potatoes, salt and water to cover. Bring to a boil over medium-high heat. Cook for 18 minutes or until tender; drain. Add margarine. Cook for several minutes longer, shaking saucepan. Add parsley; toss to coat. Makes 6 servings.

Approx. per serving: 124.0 calories; 3.8 gr. fat; 27.58% calories from fat.

TWICE-BAKED SPINACH POTATOES

You can stuff a baked potato with practically anything you can find in the refrigerator. Try mushrooms, crab meat or chili peppers.

4 medium baking potatoes, baked and cut into halves
¼ cup 1% low-fat milk
2½ teaspoons fresh lemon juice
¼ teaspoon pepper
1 pound fresh spinach, cooked and drained
Dash of paprika

Scoop out potato pulp. In a medium bowl combine potato pulp, milk, lemon juice and pepper; mash until smooth. Add spinach; mix well. Into potato shells spoon spinach mixture. Sprinkle with paprika. Preheat broiler. Broil for 10 minutes. Makes 4 servings.

Approx. per serving: 146.0 calories; 0.4 gr. fat; 2.46% calories from fat.

ORIENTAL SNOW PEA STIR-FRY

¼ cup chicken broth, either homemade or canned
1 teaspoon cornstarch
1 or 2 cloves garlic, minced
2 cups fresh snow peas
1 can (8 ounces) sliced bamboo shoots, drained
1 can (8 ounces) sliced water chestnuts, drained
2 teaspoons lite soy sauce

In a small bowl combine chicken broth and cornstarch; mix well. Set aside. Coat a nonstick skillet with vegetable cooking spray. Heat the skillet over low heat. To the heated skillet add garlic. Sauté until light brown. Add snow peas, bamboo shoots, water chestnuts and soy sauce. Increase heat. Stir-fry over high heat for 1 minute. Reduce heat to medium. Stir in the broth mixture. Bring to a boil. Cook for 1 minute or until thickened, stirring constantly. Makes 4 servings.

Approx. per serving: 66.0 calories; 0.4 gr. fat; 5.45% calories from fat.

Vegetables

CREAMED SPINACH BAKE

Spinach casserole is so pretty that its wonderful taste seems like an extra bonus. It's also a surprisingly easy recipe to prepare. Don't cook spinach in aluminum—the spinach picks up an acidic taste and becomes gray in color.

1 ½ pounds fresh spinach,
   cooked, drained and chopped
1 egg,* beaten
2 teaspoons corn oil margarine
1 tablespoon broth, either
   homemade or canned
½ cup scallions, chopped
½ cup fresh mushrooms, chopped
½ cup carrots, grated
2 tablespoons unbleached flour
¾ cup evaporated skim milk
½ teaspoon salt (optional)
¼ teaspoon pepper
¼ teaspoon nutmeg

Preheat oven to 350 degrees. In a bowl combine spinach and egg; mix well with a fork. In a skillet heat margarine and broth over medium heat. Add scallions. Sauté until tender but not brown. Add mushrooms and carrots. Cook over low heat for 5 minutes or until liquid evaporates. Add flour; stir until vegetables are coated. Add evaporated milk. Bring to a boil over medium heat, stirring constantly; reduce heat. Cook for 2 to 3 minutes, stirring constantly. Remove from heat. Stir in spinach mixture. Add salt, pepper and nutmeg. Spray a loaf pan with vegetable cooking spray. Into the prepared pan spoon the spinach mixture. Bake for 25 minutes or until firm. Cut into squares. Makes 4 servings.

* To reduce fat and cholesterol, use an egg substitute with less than 2 grams fat per serving. Fat and calorie content may vary between brands.

Approx. per serving: 118.0 calories; 3.7 gr. fat; 28.22% calories from fat.

SNOW PEAS AND TOMATOES

1 tablespoon corn oil margarine
¼ cup onion, chopped
1 pound fresh snow peas, trimmed
1 tablespoon lite soy sauce
1 teaspoon fresh oregano or
   ½ teaspoon dried oregano
3 medium tomatoes, cut into
   wedges

In a skillet over medium heat melt margarine. Add onion. Sauté until tender. Add snow peas, soy sauce and oregano. Stir-fry for about 3 minutes or until tender-crisp. Add tomatoes; cover. Cook for 1 minute longer. Into a serving dish spoon vegetables. Makes 6 servings.

Approx. per serving: 47.66 calories; 0.96 gr. fat; 18.0% calories from fat.

SPINACH OMELET

1 package (10 ounces) frozen
  chopped spinach, thawed,
  undrained
3 tablespoons chicken broth,
  either homemade or canned
1 clove garlic, crushed
1/8 to 1/4 teaspoon pepper
1/4 cup Parmesan cheese, grated
2 1/2 cups egg substitute *
2 tablespoons water
2 teaspoons corn oil margarine,
  divided

In a small saucepan over medium heat combine spinach, broth, garlic and pepper; cover. Simmer for 20 minutes. Add cheese. Cook for 1 minute or until cheese melts, stirring constantly. Set aside. In a bowl combine Egg Beaters and water; beat lightly. Spray a 10-inch omelet pan or heavy skillet with vegetable cooking spray. Add margarine. Place over medium heat until just hot enough to sizzle a drop of water. Into the heated skillet pour half the Egg Beater mixture. With a spatula lift the edges of the mixture gently as mixture starts to set so uncooked mixture flows underneath. Cook until set. Over half the omelet spread half the spinach mixture. Loosen with spatula; fold omelet over. Onto a warm serving plate slide the omelet. Repeat with the remaining margarine, Egg Beater mixture and spinach mixture. Makes 6 servings.

* Nutritional analysis based on using *Fleischmann's Egg Beaters* egg substitute. Fat and calorie content may vary between brands.

Approx. per serving: 205.0 calories; 13.8 gr. fat; 60.58% calories from fat; high vitamin A.

SPINACH ROCKEFELLER

4 pounds fresh spinach, cooked,
  drained and chopped
4 eggs *
1/2 cup dry bread crumbs
1/2 cup scallions, minced
1/4 cup Parmesan cheese,
  freshly grated
2 tablespoons corn oil margarine,
  melted
2 teaspoons fresh thyme or
  1 teaspoon dried thyme
1/2 teaspoon black pepper
1/2 teaspoon cayenne pepper
1/2 teaspoon salt (optional)
12 thick (1/4 inch each) tomato
  slices
1/2 teaspoon garlic powder

Preheat oven to 350 degrees. In a large bowl combine spinach, eggs, bread crumbs, scallions, cheese, margarine, thyme, black pepper, cayenne pepper and salt; mix well. In a shallow baking dish arrange tomato slices in a single layer. Onto each tomato slice spoon 1/4 cup spinach mixture. Sprinkle with garlic powder. Bake for 15 minutes or until spinach is set. Arrange on serving platter. Garnish with tomato slice halves if desired. Makes 12 servings.

* To reduce fat and cholesterol, use an egg substitute with less than 2 grams fat per serving. Fat and calorie content may vary between brands.

Approx. per serving: 103.0 calories; 4.3 gr. fat; 37.0% calories from fat; high vitamin A.

APPLE AND CRANBERRY ACORN SQUASH

Acorn squash is green acorn-shaped squash patched with orange. The texture is best when baked. This recipe may be made quickly in the microwave oven—just cover and microwave for 13 minutes.

**4 small acorn squash
2 medium apples, unpeeled, chopped
½ cup fresh cranberries
¼ cup packed light brown sugar
2 tablespoons almonds, chopped
1 tablespoon Grand Marnier or fresh orange juice
1 tablespoon corn oil margarine, melted**

Preheat oven to 375 degrees. Cut squash lengthwise into halves; discard seed. In a baking dish arrange squash cut side down. Add ½ inch water to dish. Bake for 40 minutes. In a bowl combine apples, cranberries, brown sugar, almonds, Grand Marnier and margarine; mix well. Turn the squash cut side up. Spoon the apple mixture into the squash cavities. Bake for 30 minutes. Makes 8 servings.

Approx. per serving: 129.0 calories; 2.8 gr. fat; 19.53% calories from fat.

BUTTERNUT SQUASH WITH GINGER AND LEMON

Buy butternut squash or other winter squash (acorn, buttercup, hubbard or pumpkin) that are hard, heavy and clean. The hard skins protect the pulp inside so squash can be stored at a cool room temperature for 3 to 4 months before eating.

**2 butternut squash (2 pounds each) or other winter squash
1 tablespoon corn oil margarine
1 tablespoon fresh gingerroot, grated
1 tablespoon fresh lemon rind, grated
Salt and freshly ground pepper to taste**

Preheat oven to 350 degrees. Puncture several holes in each squash. On a baking sheet place squash. Bake for 1 hour or until tender, turning once. Cut squash in half; discard seed, scoop out pulp and discard peel. Into a food processor container or mixer bowl place the squash pulp. Add margarine, ginger, lemon rind, salt and pepper. Process or beat just until mixed. Into a serving dish spoon the squash mixture. Serve immediately. Makes 8 servings.

Approx. per serving: 45.0 calories; 1.5 gr. fat; 30.0% calories from fat.

BOURBON ORANGE SWEET POTATOES

Use leftover mashed sweet potatoes in place of fresh mashed pumpkin in cakes, bread and cookie recipes, or try combining sweet potatoes with mashed rutabaga or turnips.

**4 pounds sweet potatoes,
   unpeeled**
⅓ cup 1% low-fat milk
¼ cup Bourbon
¼ cup fresh orange juice
¼ cup packed light brown sugar
1 tablespoon corn oil margarine
½ teaspoon salt (optional)
½ teaspoon pumpkin pie spice
¼ cup pecans, chopped

In a large saucepan over medium heat combine sweet potatoes and water to cover. Cook until tender; drain and cool. Preheat oven to 350 degrees. Peel sweet potatoes. Into a large mixer bowl place the sweet potatoes; mash. Add milk, Bourbon, orange juice, brown sugar, margarine, salt and pumpkin pie spice; beat until fluffy. Spray a baking dish with vegetable cooking spray. Into the prepared dish spoon the sweet potato mixture. Sprinkle pecans over the top. Bake for 40 minutes. Makes 8 servings.

Approx. per serving: 322.0 calories; 4.5 gr. fat; 12.57% calories from fat.

SWEET POTATOES WITH APPLES

Boiling peeled sweet potatoes causes a loss of texture and flavor, so be sure to bake or steam peeled potatoes. Whole sweet potatoes, pricked to prevent bursting, will cook in 8 minutes in the microwave.

**4 large sweet potatoes or yams,
   peeled and quartered**
½ cup packed light brown sugar
¼ cup fresh orange juice
2 teaspoons orange rind, grated
½ teaspoon cinnamon
**2 large tart cooking apples,
   unpeeled, sliced**
**2 tablespoons corn oil margarine,
   chilled and cut into
   small pieces**

In a steamer over medium heat steam sweet potatoes for 15 minutes or just until tender. Cool slightly. Cut into ½-inch slices. In a small bowl combine brown sugar, orange juice, orange rind and cinnamon; mix well. Preheat oven to 350 degrees. In a baking dish layer sweet potatoes, apples and brown sugar mixture ⅓ at a time. Dot with margarine. Bake for 30 minutes or until apples are tender. Makes 8 servings.

Approx. per serving: 159.0 calories; 3.1 gr. fat; 17.54% calories from fat.

SWEET POTATO AND APPLE CASSEROLE

3 large Granny Smith or Golden
  Delicious apples, peeled, halved,
  cored and thinly sliced
1 tablespoon fresh lemon juice
1 ½ pounds sweet potatoes,
  peeled, halved lengthwise and
  thinly sliced
¼ cup apple juice
1 tablespoon corn oil margarine,
  melted

Preheat oven to 350 degrees. In a bowl combine apples and lemon juice; toss to coat apples. Set aside the most attractive sweet potato slices. In a 1½-quart baking dish layer the remaining sweet potatoes and apples alternately. Over the layers arrange the reserved sweet potato slices in a circular overlapping pattern. Pour apple juice and margarine over top; cover. Bake for 1 hour; uncover. Bake for 15 minutes longer to brown top. Makes 6 servings.

Approx. per serving: 170.0 calories; 1.10 gr. fat; 5.8% calories from fat.

BRAISED FRESH TOMATOES

These tomatoes will keep in the refrigerator, covered, for a few days.

1 tablespoon corn oil margarine
1 ⅓ cups onions, chopped
½ cup scallions, sliced
3 pounds ripe tomatoes, peeled,
  seeded and diced
6 cloves garlic, minced
3 bay leaves
½ teaspoon salt (optional)
½ teaspoon fresh thyme or
  ¼ teaspoon dried thyme
¼ teaspoon pepper

In a skillet over medium heat melt margarine. Add onions and scallions. Sauté over medium high heat until transparent. Add tomatoes, garlic, bay leaves, salt, thyme and pepper; mix well. Bring to a boil; reduce heat. Cover. Simmer for 1 hour. Discard bay leaves. Serve hot, at room temperature or chilled. Makes 8 servings.

Approx. per serving: 56.0 calories; 1.9 gr. fat; 30.53% calories from fat.

CHERRY TOMATOES WITH PARSLEY AND GARLIC

A colorful and light vegetable dish, this goes well with almost any entrée in the book. You can serve this as a salad also—just combine all the ingredients and serve.

2 pints cherry tomatoes
  (about 40), cut into halves
4 teaspoons fresh lemon juice
1 tablespoon olive oil
2 cloves garlic, minced
½ teaspoon salt (optional)
⅔ cup fresh parsley, coarsely
  chopped

Preheat oven to 350 degrees. In a medium baking dish combine tomatoes, lemon juice, olive oil, garlic and salt; toss lightly. Bake for 5 minutes or until heated through. Stir in parsley just before serving. Makes 8 servings.

Approx. per serving: 30.0 calories; 1.8 gr. fat; 54.0% calories from fat.

TOMATOES FLORENTINE

6 medium tomatoes
2 tablespoons corn oil margarine
1 small onion, finely chopped
1 clove garlic, minced
1 package (10 ounces) frozen
  spinach, thawed, drained and
  chopped
⅓ cup 1% low-fat milk
Salt and freshly ground pepper
  to taste
2 tablespoons fine dry bread
  crumbs
2 tablespoons fresh parsley,
  chopped
2 tablespoons Parmesan cheese,
  freshly grated

Preheat oven to 400 degrees. Slice tops off tomatoes. Scoop out half the pulp and reserve for sauce or soup. In a skillet over medium heat melt margarine. Add onion and garlic. Sauté until tender. Add spinach, milk, salt and pepper; mix well. Into tomato shells spoon spinach mixture. In an ovenproof serving dish or on a baking sheet place tomatoes. In a small bowl combine bread crumbs, parsley and cheese; mix well. Sprinkle over tomatoes. Bake for 20 minutes or until heated through. Makes 6 servings.

Approx. per serving: 73.0 calories; 2.1 gr. fat; 25.89% calories from fat.

Vegetables

TOMATO WEDGES PROVENÇAL

4 medium tomatoes, each cut into
   8 wedges
¼ cup fine bread crumbs
¼ cup onion, finely chopped
¼ cup parsley, chopped
1 clove garlic, minced
1 tablespoon corn oil margarine
½ teaspoon fresh basil or
   ¼ teaspoon dried basil
Salt and pepper to taste

Preheat oven to 425 degrees. In a greased shallow baking dish arrange tomatoes. In a small bowl combine bread crumbs, onion, parsley, garlic, margarine, basil, salt and pepper; mix well. Sprinkle over tomatoes. Bake for 8 to 10 minutes or until tender.
Makes 6 servings.

Approx. per serving: 44.5 calories; 1.04 gr. fat; 21.0% calories from fat.

SEE RED RELISH

6 large tomatoes, peeled, cored
   and chopped
6 large red bell peppers, chopped
2 large onions, chopped
1 ½ cups granulated sugar
½ cup cider vinegar
1 teaspoon cayenne pepper
½ teaspoon salt (optional)

In a large saucepan place tomatoes. Cook over low heat for 45 minutes. Add red peppers, onions, sugar, vinegar, cayenne pepper and salt; mix well. Cook until thickened.
Makes 3 cups (¼ cup per serving).

Approx. per serving: 122.0 calories; 0.38 gr. fat; 2.8% calories from fat.

SAUTÉED ZUCCHINI

Use a nonstick skillet and sauté the zucchini in just a bit of margarine and water, which evaporates as the vegetable cooks. Other vegetables can be prepared the same way.

1 teaspoon corn oil margarine
4 medium zucchini, cut into
  ¼-inch rounds
2 scallions, thinly sliced
¼ cup water

In a nonstick skillet over low heat melt the margarine. Add zucchini, scallions and water. Increase heat. Sauté over medium heat for 2 minutes. Serve immediately. Makes 8 servings.

Approx. per serving: 18.0 calories; 0.5 gr. fat; 25.0% calories from fat.

ZUCCHINI À LA GRÈCQUE

8 small zucchini, scored
  lengthwise with fork
⅔ cup water
1 tablespoon corn oil margarine
1 medium onion, chopped
1 clove garlic, chopped
4 ripe tomatoes, peeled and
  chopped
Salt and pepper to taste

In a large saucepan combine zucchini and water. Cook over medium heat for 6 minutes or until tender. Remove from heat; set aside. In a medium skillet heat margarine over medium heat. Add onion and garlic. Sauté until tender. Add tomatoes. Cook until tender. Season with salt and pepper. Drain zucchini. On a serving plate arrange zucchini. Spoon tomato sauce over top. Makes 6 to 8 servings.

Approx. per serving: 52.62 calories; 1.0 gr. fat; 17.0% calories from fat.

FRESH STIR-FRY MELANGE

2 tablespoons olive oil
3½ cups fresh green bell peppers, cut into strips
3½ cups fresh red bell peppers, cut into strips
2½ cups fresh mushrooms, sliced
1 cup celery, sliced
2 tablespoons onion, chopped
¾ teaspoon salt (optional)
½ clove garlic, crushed
½ teaspoon granulated sugar
½ teaspoon fresh oregano or
¼ teaspoon dried oregano
Dash of pepper
2 tomatoes, cut into wedges
1 teaspoon wine vinegar

In a skillet or wok heat olive oil over medium-high heat. Add green and red pepper strips, mushrooms, celery, onion, salt, garlic, sugar, oregano and pepper. Stir-fry until peppers are tender-crisp. Add tomatoes and vinegar. Stir-fry until heated through. Makes 6 servings.

Approx. per serving: 83.0 calories; 5.1 gr. fat; 55.3% calories from fat.

MICROWAVE GARDEN TRIO

1 tablespoon corn oil margarine
½ pound fresh asparagus spears, cut into 2-inch pieces
½ teaspoon basil
Pinch of pepper
½ pound fresh mushrooms, sliced
1 medium tomato, cut into wedges
Salt to taste

In a 1½-quart glass baking dish microwave margarine on High for 30 seconds. Add asparagus, basil and pepper; mix well. Cover. Microwave for 3 minutes. Add mushrooms; cover. Microwave for 3 minutes. Add tomato; cover. Microwave for 1½ minutes longer. Season with salt; cover. Let stand for 3 minutes. Makes 4 servings.

Approx. per serving: 72.75 calories; 1.79 gr. fat; 22.0% calories from fat.

GARDEN RATATOUILLE

Eggplant originated in tropical Asia and was gradually adopted by Near Eastern and Mediterranean cuisines, where it is now very much at home. This colorful blend from the south of France is good hot or cold and is excellent combined with pasta.

2 small eggplant, peeled and
  thinly sliced
Salt to taste
2 tablespoons olive oil, divided
4 small zucchini, sliced
2 cups onions, chopped
3 cloves garlic, minced
3 green bell peppers, cut into
  cubes
2 cups fresh tomatoes, chopped
½ cup fresh parsley, chopped
2 teaspoons fresh oregano or
  1 teaspoon dried oregano
½ teaspoon granulated sugar
½ teaspoon salt (optional)
¼ teaspoon pepper
6 cups cooked brown rice

Preheat oven to 325 degrees. In a colander sprinkle eggplant with salt. Drain for 30 minutes. Dry with paper towels. Brush a nonstick skillet with a small amount of oil. In the oiled skillet sauté the eggplant over medium heat until softened, brushing skillet with oil as necessary. Remove eggplant. Add the remaining oil and zucchini. Sauté until tender. Remove zucchini with a slotted spoon. Add onions and garlic. Sauté for 5 minutes. Add green peppers, tomatoes, parsley, oregano, sugar, ½ teaspoon salt and pepper. Cook for 5 minutes longer. In a casserole layer eggplant, zucchini and tomato mixture ½ at a time; cover. Bake for 1 hour. Serve over hot rice. Makes 8 servings.

Approx. per serving: 270.0 calories; 4.9 gr. fat; 16.33% calories from fat.

RATATOUILLE PIZZA

1 tablespoon corn oil or
  safflower oil
1½ teaspoons Italian seasoning
2 cups eggplant, chopped
1 cup zucchini, thinly sliced
1 medium green bell pepper,
  cut into 1-inch squares
1 medium tomato, peeled and
  chopped
½ cup onion, chopped
1 clove garlic, minced
1 loaf Italian bread, cut in half
  lengthwise
1½ cups part-skim mozzarella
  cheese, divided

Preheat oven to 375 degrees. In a large skillet heat oil and Italian seasoning over medium heat. Add eggplant, zucchini, green pepper, tomato, onion and garlic. Sauté until tender-crisp. Reduce heat. Simmer for 5 minutes. On a baking sheet place bread. Sprinkle ½ cup cheese on bread. Spoon sautéed vegetables over cheese. Bake for 10 minutes or until edges brown. Sprinkle with the remaining cheese. Bake for 3 to 5 minutes longer or until cheese is melted. Makes 8 servings.

Approx. per serving: 249.0 calories; 5.3 gr. fat; 19.15% calories from fat.

TEX-MEX
STIR-FRY

2 tablespoons corn oil or
  safflower oil
¾ cup onion, coarsely chopped
¾ cup green bell pepper,
  coarsely chopped
1 clove garlic, finely minced
1½ cups tomatoes, cored and
  cut into ½-inch cubes
¾ cup water
1 tablespoon chili powder
½ teaspoon cumin, ground
3 cups zucchini, diced
¾ teaspoon salt (optional)
1 cup fresh or frozen corn

In a large skillet heat oil over medium-high heat. Add onion, green pepper and garlic. Sauté for 5 minutes or until onion is tender. Add tomatoes, water, chili powder and cumin. Bring to a boil. Reduce heat to low; cover. Simmer for 5 minutes. Add zucchini and salt. Simmer for 5 to 8 minutes or until zucchini is tender. Stir in corn. Simmer for 1 minute longer. Makes 4 servings.

Approx. per serving: 148.0 calories; 4.46 gr. fat; 27.0% calories from fat.

VEGETABLE
CUSTARD

1 cup whole wheat bread crumbs
2 tablespoons corn oil margarine,
  melted
1 cup zucchini, sliced
1 cup fresh mushrooms, sliced
1 cup fresh green beans
1 cup carrots, sliced
1 cup onion, chopped
½ cup green bell pepper, chopped
2 cups 1% low-fat milk
4 eggs, * well beaten
Salt and pepper to taste
Nutmeg to taste
1 tomato, sliced
2 tablespoons Parmesan cheese,
  freshly grated

Preheat oven to 375 degrees. Grease an 8-inch springform pan. In the prepared pan sprinkle bread crumbs. In a medium skillet heat 1 tablespoon margarine over medium heat. Add zucchini, mushrooms, green beans, carrots, onion and green pepper. Sauté until vegetables are tender-crisp. Into the prepared pan spoon vegetables. In a medium bowl beat milk, eggs, salt, pepper and nutmeg. Pour over sautéed vegetables. Arrange tomato slices over top. Sprinkle with Parmesan cheese and the remaining 1 tablespoon melted margarine. Bake for 25 minutes or until set. On a serving plate place springform pan; remove side of pan. Cut custard into wedges. Makes 8 servings.

* To reduce fat and cholesterol, use an egg substitute with less than 2 grams fat per serving. Fat and calorie content may vary between brands.

Approx. per serving: 182.0 calories; 8.2 gr. fat; 40.54% calories from fat; high vitamin A.

VEGETABLE STEW

This wonderful dish from the south of France will come to the table in a burst of color and aroma. The vegetables that take longest to cook go into the pot first, the most tender last so each is prepared perfectly.

16 small fresh pearl onions
1 ½ cups (about) water, divided
1 teaspoon fresh thyme or
½ teaspoon dried thyme
1 teaspoon fresh tarragon or
½ teaspoon dried tarragon
Salt (optional)
12 carrots, peeled and cut into
2-inch pieces
½ small bunch broccoli, cut into
florets
½ small cauliflower, cut into
florets
6 summer squash, cut into
2-inch pieces
4 small zucchini, halved
lengthwise
24 green beans, trimmed and
cut into 2-inch pieces
1 tablespoon mixed fresh basil,
parsley, thyme and tarragon or
1 teaspoon mixed dried herbs
2 cloves garlic, finely chopped
3 tablespoons olive oil
Freshly ground pepper to taste

Bring a large saucepan of salted water to a boil. Maintain the boil while cooking the vegetables. In a large sauté pan over medium heat combine the onions, 1 cup water, 1 teaspoon thyme, 1 teaspoon tarragon and a pinch of salt; cover. Simmer for 5 minutes. Into the saucepan place the carrots. Cook for 2 minutes; remove carrots to the sauté pan. Cover. Simmer the onions and carrots for 5 minutes. Into the boiling water place the broccoli and cauliflower. Cook for 5 minutes; remove to the sauté pan. Add ½ cup water; toss to mix and cover. Continue simmering.

Add the squash and zucchini to the boiling water. Cook for 3 minutes; remove to the sauté pan. Add green beans to the boiling water. Cook for 1 minute. Remove the beans to the sauté pan. Toss the vegetables together; add water if necessary. Liquid should equal about 1 cup. Cover. Cook for 5 minutes. Uncover; turn heat to high. Add mixed herbs, garlic and olive oil. Cook until sauce thickens slightly, tossing vegetables constantly. Add salt and pepper to taste. Makes 8 servings.

Approx. per serving: 128.75 calories; 5.69 gr. fat; 40.0% calories from fat.

VEGETABLE DELLA ROBBIA

2 pounds fresh broccoli, trimmed
Florets of 1 small head cauliflower
1 carrot, peeled and thinly sliced
1 zucchini, sliced ¼ inch thick
4 ounces fresh mushrooms, sliced
1 small red bell pepper, cut into
wide strips
2 tablespoons corn oil margarine,
melted

On a microwave-safe platter arrange broccoli with stems toward center. Place cauliflower florets in center of platter. Around the cauliflower arrange carrot, zucchini and mushrooms. Arrange red pepper strips in flower design over cauliflower. Drizzle with margarine; cover with plastic wrap. Microwave on High for 10 to 12 minutes or until vegetables are tender, turning platter every 4 minutes. Let stand for 5 minutes. Serve with Parmesan cheese if desired. Makes 8 servings.

Approx. per serving: 77.0 calories; 3.5 gr. fat; 40.0% calories from fat.

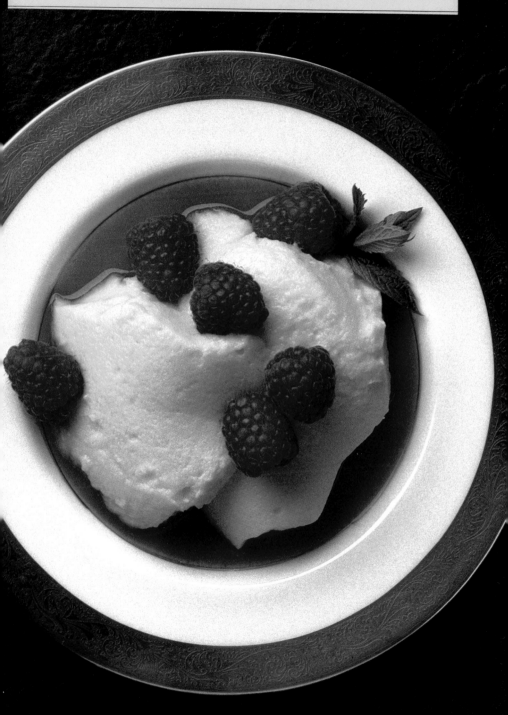

We offer some imaginative desserts to please dessert lovers while staying within the bounds of good nutrition. All are low in fat and many are based on fruit. Skim milk, low-fat cottage cheese and yogurt are often used in place of cream.

For those of you who are still tempted by high-fat, low-nutrition desserts, perhaps this information will bring you back in line. A slice of pecan pie provides 460 calories and 40% of the fat requirement for a day. Two scoops of ice cream can provide two-thirds of your day's fat allowance.

As an alternative, look for nonfat low-calorie fruit yogurt or add your own fresh fruit to nonfat low-calorie yogurt.

An American Cancer Society study on the use of artificial sweeteners had interesting results. The study showed those who used artificial sweeteners gained more weight than those who did not. Apparently, people using artificial sweeteners tended to eat more fattening foods, because they felt they had compensated by not using sugar. In fact, sugar has only 16 calories a teaspoon, and the actual calories saved are minimal. Also, adding artificial creamer to coffee adds 35 calories of the most saturated fat—coconut oil. Use 1% low-fat or skim milk as a substitute.

Recipe for this photograph on page 199.

BUTTERMILK CHOCOLATE DROPS

This is a no-fail recipe, even for a novice cook.

1 cup packed light brown sugar
½ cup shortening
4 squares (1 ounce each) unsweetened chocolate, melted
1 egg *
1 teaspoon vanilla extract
1¾ cups all-purpose flour
2 teaspoons baking powder
½ teaspoon baking soda
¼ teaspoon salt (optional)
½ cup buttermilk

Preheat oven to 350 degrees. In a mixer bowl cream brown sugar and shortening until light and fluffy. Add chocolate, egg and vanilla; mix well. In a small bowl combine flour, baking powder, baking soda and salt; mix lightly. To the creamed mixture add the dry ingredients alternately with buttermilk, mixing well after each addition. Grease cookie sheets lightly or use nonstick cookie sheets. Onto the prepared cookie sheets drop dough by teaspoonfuls. Bake for 12 to 15 minutes or until brown.
Makes 5 dozen cookies.

* To reduce fat and cholesterol, use an egg substitute with less than 2 grams fat per serving. Fat and calorie content may vary between brands.

Approx. per cookie: 54.0 calories; 2.86 gr. fat; 47.66% calories from fat.

CRACKER JACK COOKIES

These cookies are guaranteed to disappear, probably before they are even cooled!

1 cup corn oil margarine, softened
1 cup packed light brown sugar
1 cup granulated sugar
2 eggs *
2 teaspoons vanilla extract
1½ cups all-purpose flour
1 teaspoon baking powder
1 teaspoon baking soda
½ teaspoon salt (optional)
2 cups rolled oats
2 cups crispy rice cereal
1 cup coconut, flaked

Preheat oven to 350 degrees. In a large mixer bowl cream margarine, brown sugar and granulated sugar until light and fluffy. Add eggs and vanilla; mix well. In a small bowl combine flour, baking powder, baking soda and salt; mix lightly. To the creamed mixture add dry ingredients; mix well. Stir in oats, cereal and coconut. Grease cookie sheets or use nonstick cookie sheets. Onto the prepared cookie sheets drop dough by teaspoonfuls. Bake for 10 to 12 minutes or until brown.
Makes 6 to 7 dozen cookies.

* To reduce fat and cholesterol, use an egg substitute with less than 2 grams fat per serving. Fat and calorie content may vary between brands.

Approx. per cookie: 64.0 calories; 2.9 gr. fat; 40.78% calories from fat.

OATMEAL-CARROT BARS

This recipe makes a good after-school or lunch box treat.

¾ cup packed light brown sugar
¼ cup corn oil margarine, softened
1 egg *
1½ to 2 cups carrots, shredded
1 teaspoon vanilla extract
1 cup whole wheat flour
1 teaspoon baking powder
1 teaspoon cinnamon
¼ teaspoon salt (optional)
½ to ¾ cup uncooked oats
½ cup raisins
2 tablespoons wheat germ

Preheat oven to 350 degrees. In a large mixer bowl cream brown sugar, margarine and egg until light and fluffy. Add carrots and vanilla; mix well. In a small bowl combine whole wheat flour, baking powder, cinnamon and salt. To creamed mixture add dry ingredients; mix well. Stir in oats, raisins and wheat germ. Lightly grease a 9-inch square baking pan. In prepared pan spread batter. Bake for 30 minutes or until set in center. Cool. Cut into squares. Makes 2 dozen squares.

* To reduce fat and cholesterol, use an egg substitute with less than 2 grams fat per serving. Fat and calorie content may vary between brands.

Approx. per square: 88.6 calories; 2.7 gr. fat; 27.42% calories from fat.

HIKER'S HONEY FRUIT SQUARES

These cookies keep well and stay moist and chewy "on the trail."

2 eggs *
¾ cup honey
½ cup all-purpose flour
½ cup graham cracker crumbs
1 cup currants or dates, chopped or prunes, pitted and chopped
½ cup nuts, chopped

Preheat oven to 350 degrees. Grease and flour an 8-inch square baking pan. In a medium mixer bowl beat eggs until very light. Add honey gradually in a very fine stream, beating constantly. Stir in flour and graham cracker crumbs. Add currants and nuts; mix well. In the prepared baking pan spread batter. Bake for 30 to 40 minutes or until firm in center and brown on top. Cool. Cut into squares. Makes 16 squares.

* To reduce fat and cholesterol, use an egg substitute with less than 2 grams fat per serving. Fat and calorie content may vary between brands.

Approx. per square: 168.0 calories; 3.3 gr. fat; 17.67% calories from fat.

PINEAPPLE-ORANGE BARS

This no-bake dessert is perfect to make on hot summer days.

⅔ cup plus 2 tablespoons graham cracker crumbs, divided
2 tablespoons corn oil margarine
½ cup instant nonfat dry milk powder
½ cup unsweetened fresh orange juice, chilled
1 egg white
1 tablespoon fresh lemon juice
¼ cup granulated sugar
1 can (8 ounces) unsweetened crushed pineapple, drained

In a small bowl combine ⅔ cup graham cracker crumbs and margarine; mix well. Press mixture into an 8-inch square dish; set aside. In a large mixer bowl combine dry milk powder, orange juice, egg white and lemon juice. Beat at high speed of electric mixer for 3 minutes. Add sugar. Beat for 3 minutes longer. Fold in pineapple gently. Into the prepared dish spoon the pineapple mixture. Sprinkle the remaining 2 tablespoons graham cracker crumbs on top. Freeze for 8 hours to overnight. Let stand at room temperature for 15 minutes before serving. Makes 9 servings.

Approx. per serving: 115.0 calories; 3.4 gr. fat; 26.6% calories from fat.

CANTALOUPE ICE

Using this same simple procedure, there is an endless variety of fruits and juices that can be transformed into a refreshing dessert. The best fruits for sorbets are very ripe cantaloupes or other melons, mangoes, pears, raspberries, strawberries, blueberries and blackberries.

1½ cups water
½ cup granulated sugar
2 very ripe cantaloupes, cut into halves and seeded
¼ cup fresh lemon juice

In a small saucepan combine water and sugar. Bring to a boil over medium-high heat. Reduce heat. Simmer for 5 minutes; cool. Into a blender container or food processor scoop cantaloupe pulp and juice. Add lemon juice and cooled syrup. Purée until smooth. Pour into mixer bowl. Freeze until partially frozen. Beat with electric mixer until smooth. Spoon into freezer container; cover. Freeze until firm. Let stand at room tem-

perature for several minutes. Into dessert glasses spoon Cantaloupe Ice. Makes 6 servings.

Approx. per serving: 139.0 calories; 0.6 gr. fat; 3.88% calories from fat.

CHOCOLATE MOUSSE

This is our low-fat adaptation of this French favorite. We know you will find it extraordinary.

1 large egg *
1 tablespoon cold water
1 envelope unflavored gelatin
1 cup boiling water
½ cup part-skim ricotta cheese
½ cup cold 1% low-fat milk
¼ cup plus 2 tablespoons granulated sugar
1½ tablespoons unsweetened cocoa powder
1 teaspoon instant coffee powder
Pinch of salt (optional)
6 whole fresh strawberries

In a blender container or food processor combine egg, cold water and gelatin. Process for 10 seconds. Scrape sides. Process for 10 seconds longer. Let stand for 1 minute or until gelatin is softened. Add boiling water. Process for 10 seconds or until gelatin is dissolved. Add ricotta cheese, milk, sugar, cocoa, coffee powder and salt. Process for 1 minute. Into 6 dessert cups pour mousse. Chill for 2 hours or until set. Garnish with a strawberry. Makes 6 servings.

* To reduce fat and cholesterol, use an egg substitute with less than 2 grams fat per serving. Fat and calorie content may vary between brands.

Approx. per serving: 124.0 calories; 5.3 gr. fat; 38.46% calories from fat.

LIGHT ORANGE CHEESECAKE

Rich, creamy, luscious cheesecakes are what dieters dream about. Our slimmed-down version lets you have your cake and eat it too—without guilt. It is made with all natural ingredients—no sugar substitutes to make it taste "low-calorie"—, and it is tasty enough to be enjoyed by those not counting calories as well. So satisfy your passion for America's favorite dessert and dig in. But, remember, only one piece!

**1½ cups fresh orange juice,
  divided
2 envelopes unflavored gelatin
3 cups low-fat cottage cheese
¾ cup granulated sugar, divided
2 eggs, separated
1 teaspoon orange rind,
  freshly grated
1 teaspoon vanilla extract
⅛ teaspoon salt (optional)
¼ cup graham cracker crumbs**

In a small bowl place ½ cup orange juice. Sprinkle gelatin on top. Let stand until softened. In a small saucepan over medium-high heat bring remaining 1 cup orange juice to a boil. Add to gelatin mixture; stir until gelatin dissolves. Into a blender or a food processor fitted with metal blade pour orange juice mixture. Add cottage cheese, ½ cup sugar, egg yolks, orange rind, vanilla and salt. Process until smooth. Into a large bowl pour the cottage cheese mixture. Chill until mixture mounds slightly when dropped from a spoon. In a mixer bowl beat egg whites until soft peaks form. Add remaining ¼ cup sugar gradually, beating constantly until stiff peaks form. Into the orange mixture fold the egg whites gently. Over the bottom of an 8-inch springform cake pan sprinkle crumbs. Spoon orange mixture carefully over crumbs. Chill until firm. Onto a serving plate place cheesecake. Remove side of pan. Serve with fresh berries. Makes 12 servings.

Approx. per serving: 135.0 calories; 2.2 gr. fat; 14.66% calories from fat.

CITRUS CHEESECAKE

Our version of the ever popular, but too rich cheesecake will please cheesecake lovers with its lemon and orange-scented flavor and its luscious creamy texture.

**⅔ cup cornflakes
¼ cup Grape Nuts
2 teaspoons corn oil margarine,
  melted
2 teaspoons fresh lemon rind,
  grated, divided
1 teaspoon fresh orange rind,
  grated
1 teaspoon light brown sugar
2 envelopes unflavored gelatin
¾ cup granulated sugar, divided
1½ cups 1% low-fat milk
3 eggs, separated
3 cups ricotta cheese
1 tablespoon fresh orange juice
1 tablespoon fresh lemon juice
1 teaspoon vanilla extract
2 kiwifruit, peeled and sliced**

Preheat oven to 350 degrees. In a blender container or food processor combine cornflakes and Grape Nuts. Process until crushed. In a medium bowl combine crushed cereals, margarine, 1 teaspoon lemon rind, orange rind and brown sugar; mix well. Over the bottom of an 8-inch springform pan press the cereal mixture. Bake for 5 minutes. Cool. In the top of a double boiler combine ¼ cup sugar and gelatin. Stir in milk and egg yolks. Let stand until gelatin softens. In the bottom of the double

boiler place a small amount of water. Heat water over low heat until simmering. Over the hot water place the top of the double boiler. Cook until the mixture coats a spoon, stirring constantly. Chill until partially set. In a food processor process ricotta cheese until smooth. In a medium bowl combine the ricotta cheese with orange juice, lemon juice, remaining 1 teaspoon lemon rind and vanilla; mix well. Fold in the partially congealed mixture gently. In a mixer bowl beat the egg whites until foamy. Add the remaining ½ cup sugar gradually, beating constantly until soft peaks form. Into the ricotta mixture fold the egg whites gently. Into the prepared pan pour the mixture. Chill for 8 hours or longer. On a serving plate place pan; remove side. Arrange kiwifruit on top.
Makes 12 servings.

Approx. per serving: 196.0 calories; 7.3 gr. fat; 33.52% calories from fat.

ORANGES
MARSALA

This dessert is icy cold, bright and refreshing. Refrigerate for at least four hours.

8 oranges
1 cup granulated sugar
½ cup Marsala
½ cup water
Juice of 1 lemon

With a vegetable peeler cut a thin layer of rind (zest) from oranges; cut into thin strips. Peel oranges completely; discard peel and set oranges aside. In a saucepan combine the orange zest, sugar, Marsala, water and lemon juice. Bring to a boil over medium-high heat; reduce heat. Simmer

until reduced by ⅓. Cool. In a bowl place whole oranges. Pour syrup over oranges. Refrigerate for several hours, basting frequently with syrup. Serve cold.
Makes 8 servings.

Approx. per serving: 176.0 calories; 1.6 gr. fat; 8.18% calories from fat.

PEACH AND
BLUEBERRY CRISP

It's hard to find a better-tasting summer fruit dessert than this one. If you cook it in a microwave, it takes only 10 minutes.

6 cups fresh peaches, peeled and sliced
2 cups fresh blueberries
⅓ cup plus ¼ cup packed light brown sugar, divided
2 tablespoons all-purpose flour
1 tablespoon cinnamon, divided
1 cup quick-cooking oats
3 tablespoons corn oil margarine

Preheat oven to 350 degrees if not using microwave. In a 2-quart baking dish or microwave-safe dish combine peaches and blueberries. In a small bowl combine ⅓ cup brown sugar, flour and 2 teaspoons cinnamon; mix well. Add to peaches and blueberries; toss to mix. In a bowl combine oats, remaining ¼ cup brown sugar and 1 teaspoon cinnamon. With a pastry blender cut in margarine until crumbly. Sprinkle over the fruit. Bake for 25 minutes or microwave on High for 10 minutes or until fruit is just tender and mixture is bubbly. Serve warm or cold. Makes 8 servings.

Approx. per serving: 203.0 calories; 5.0 gr. fat; 22.16% calories from fat.

KEY LIME YOGURT PIE

A variation of the Key West specialty, our filling is sweetened with apple juice concentrate and flavored with Key limes.

1¼ cups graham cracker crumbs
2 tablespoons corn oil margarine, melted
½ cup frozen apple juice concentrate, thawed
1 envelope unflavored gelatin
⅓ cup granulated sugar
⅓ cup fresh lime juice
2 teaspoons lime rind, freshly grated
¼ teaspoon vanilla extract
1½ cups low-fat plain yogurt
Fresh lime slices

In a small bowl combine crumbs and margarine; mix well. Over bottom and side of a pie plate press the crumb mixture. Freeze. Into a saucepan pour apple juice. Sprinkle with gelatin. Let stand for several minutes or until gelatin is softened. Add sugar. Cook over low heat until gelatin and sugar dissolve, stirring constantly. Into a mixer bowl pour the gelatin mixture. Add lime juice and rind and vanilla. Chill until the mixture resembles raw egg whites. Beat until fluffy. Add yogurt; beat until fluffy. Into the prepared crust pour the yogurt mixture. Chill until firm. Garnish with lime slices. Makes 6 to 8 servings.

Approx. per serving: 152.0 calories; 4.6 gr. fat; 27.23% calories from fat.

POACHED PEARS WITH STRAWBERRY SAUCE

Bartlett, Bosc, or Anjou pears will be superb gently simmered in syrup and spices and then coated with a bright red strawberry sauce.

4 large ripe pears, peeled and cored
4 cups apple juice
2 tablespoons granulated sugar
1 stick cinnamon
1 teaspoon orange rind, freshly grated
½ teaspoon lemon rind, freshly grated
¼ teaspoon cloves, ground
Strawberry Sauce (see page 77)
Fresh mint leaves

From bottom of each pear cut a small slice so pears will sit upright. In a large saucepan combine apple juice, sugar, cinnamon, orange rind, lemon rind and cloves. Bring to a boil over medium heat; reduce heat. Simmer for 5 minutes. Add pears; cover. Poach for 20 minutes or until pears are tender. Let stand in poaching liquid until cool. Refrigerate until serving time. To dessert plates remove pears with a slotted spoon. Drizzle Strawberry Sauce over pears. Garnish with mint leaves. Makes 4 servings.

Approx. per serving: 121.0 calories; 0.7 gr. fat; 5.2% calories from fat.

FRESH STRAWBERRY SORBET

Fresh, ripe strawberries make a delicious easy-to-make sorbet. Serve with other fruit ices or sorbets and fresh fruit.

1 cup water
1 cup granulated sugar
4 cups fresh ripe strawberries, washed and hulled
Juice of 2 oranges
Juice of 1 lemon
8 fresh whole strawberries

In a saucepan combine water and sugar. Bring to a boil over medium-high heat, stirring until sugar dissolves. Boil for 2 minutes. Cool. In a food processor or blender container purée strawberries. In a bowl combine the sugar syrup, strawberry purée, orange juice and lemon juice; mix well. Pour into ice cream freezer. Freeze according to manufacturer's instructions. (Or pour sorbet mixture into metal pan or bowl. Place in freezer. Freeze until hard then process in food processor until mixture is a hard slush. Or freeze just until firm then beat by hand or with electric mixer until slushy. Into the pan or bowl spoon slush. Freeze until firm.) Sorbet should not be served rock-hard. Transfer to refrigerator 15 minutes before serving or process in food processor. Into 8 individual stemmed glasses spoon sorbet. Garnish each with a fresh strawberry. Makes 8 servings.

Approx. per serving: 121.0 calories; 0.3 gr. fat; 2.23% calories from fat.

STRAWBERRY-LEMON MOUSSE

A light and refreshing strawberry mousse with a hint of lemon makes a perfect ending to a dinner.

1 cup granulated sugar, divided
½ cup cornstarch
3 cups 1% low-fat milk
½ cup fresh lemon juice
2 teaspoons lemon rind, freshly grated
4 egg whites, at room temperature
2½ cups fresh strawberries, sliced and chilled

In a medium saucepan mix ¾ cup sugar and cornstarch. Stir in milk gradually. Cook over medium heat until smooth and thickened, stirring constantly; remove from heat. Stir in lemon juice and rind. Cool, stirring occasionally. In a mixer bowl beat egg whites until foamy. Add remaining ¼ cup sugar 1 tablespoon at a time, beating until soft peaks form. Fold gently into lemon mixture. Into individual dishes spoon ½-cup portions. Chill until firm. Top each serving with ¼ cup strawberries. Makes 10 servings.

Approx. per serving: 142.0 calories; 0.27 gr. fat; 1.71% calories from fat.

Photograph for this recipe on page 191.

STRAWBERRIES CARDINAL

The brilliant color of the raspberry purée makes a bowl full of strawberries a more beautiful sight than ever.

1⅓ cups fresh strawberries, sliced
⅓ cup orange juice, freshly squeezed
½ cup fresh raspberries

In a bowl combine strawberries and orange juice. Marinate for 1 to 4 hours. In a food processor fitted with chopping blade place raspberries. Process until puréed. Through a fine sieve press purée to remove seed. Drain strawberries. Into individual dessert dishes spoon strawberries. Top with puréed raspberries. Makes 4 servings.

Approx. per serving: 31.0 calories; 0.3 gr. fat; 8.7% calories from fat.

SOPHISTICATED STRAWBERRIES

This is an outstanding, healthy, no-fat dessert.

1½ quarts fresh whole strawberries
2 cups low-fat vanilla yogurt
¼ cup Amaretto

Reserve 8 whole strawberries for garnish. Hull the remaining strawberries; cut into halves. Into sherbet glasses place strawberries. In a small bowl combine yogurt and Amaretto; blend well. Pour over strawberries in sherbet glasses. Garnish with reserved strawberries. May serve in meringue shells or on angel food cake slices. Makes 8 servings.

Approx. per serving: 89.8 calories; 0.5 gr. fat; 5.01% calories from fat.

STRAWNANA REFRESHER

The yogurt in this dessert is a delightful complement to the fruit, resulting in a sweet but refreshing end to a meal. Try this dessert with other frozen fruits or with added flavorings such as cinnamon, nutmeg, etc.

¾ cup fresh or frozen unsweetened strawberries
2 small bananas, cut up
1½ cups low-fat plain yogurt

Thaw frozen strawberries for 5 to 10 minutes. In a blender container combine strawberries, bananas and yogurt. Process until blended. Into 4 dessert dishes spoon mixture. Serve immediately or refrigerate until serving time. Makes 4 servings.

Approx. per serving: 118.0 calories; 1.6 gr. fat; 12.2% calories from fat.

INDIVIDUAL MERINGUE SHELLS

Light, crisp, sweet and easy to prepare if you make sure your utensils are clean and dry. Don't use plastic bowls for beating, and be sure there are no bits of yolk in the egg whites. This is a good way to use up leftover egg whites.

3 egg whites (⅓ to ½ cup), at room temperature
¼ teaspoon cream of tartar
¾ cup regular or superfine granulated sugar
¼ teaspoon vanilla or almond extract (optional)

Preheat oven to 225 degrees. Cover a baking sheet with baking parchment or foil. In a small mixer bowl combine egg whites and cream of tartar. Beat until foamy. Add sugar 1 tablespoon at a time and vanilla, beating constantly until stiff peaks form. Onto the prepared baking sheet drop meringue ⅓ cup at a time; shape into circles with back of spoon building up edge. Bake for 1 hour. Turn off oven. Let meringues stand in closed oven for 1 hour or longer. Peel off foil. Onto wire rack place meringues to cool completely. In an airtight container store meringues for up to 2 days or freeze for longer storage. Fill meringue shells with fresh fruit or yogurt topped with fresh fruit. Shells may also be shaped by piping meringue onto baking sheet using pastry bag fitted with large star tip. Makes 8 to 10 shells.

Approx. per shell: 73.5 calories; 0.0 gr. fat; 0.0% calories from fat.

$\mathcal{I}$ n d e x

$\mathscr{I}$ n d e x

Index

Index